PHEOCHROMOCYTOMA – A NEW VIEW OF THE OLD PROBLEM

Edited by **Jose Fernando Martin**

Pheochromocytoma – A New View of the Old Problem
Edited by Jose Fernando Martin

Published by InTech

Janeza Trdine 9, 51000 Rijeka, Croatia

Publishing Process Manager Masa Vidovic

Technical Editor Teodora Smiljanic

Cover Designer InTech Design Team

Additional hard copies can be obtained from orders@intechopen.com

Pheochromocytoma – A New View of the Old Problem, Edited by Jose Fernando Martin
p. cm.
ISBN 978-953-307-822-9

For EU product safety concerns:
IN TECH d.o.o., Prolaz Marije Krucifikse Kozulić 3, 51000 Rijeka, Croatia,
info@intechopen.com or visit our website at intechopen.com.

Meet the editor

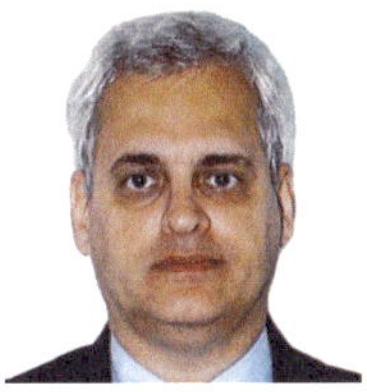

Dr. José Fernando Vilela Martin, MD, PhD is Professor of Medicine, and Head of Internal Medicine Division of State Medical School in São José do Rio Preto (FAMERP), São Paulo, Brazil. He is coordinator of Hypertension Clinic, an Experimental and Clinical Research Center associate with The National Council for Scientific and Technological Development (CNPq).He received his medical degree from FAMERP in 1986 and completed residency in Internal Medicine at University of São Paulo - Medical School in Ribeirão Preto and in Clinical Cardiology at Cardiovascular Diseases Institute in São José do Rio Preto. He completed his clinical and research training at the University of São Paulo in 1998, where he received his PhD title. Dr. Martin is a member of American Heart Association (AHA) and The Endocrine Society, besides the Brazilian Society of Hypertension, Brazilian Society of Cardiology and São Paulo Cardiological Society. He is also a reviewer on the Pan American Journal of Public Health and a scientific advisor of the Hypertension Department of Brazilian Society of Cardiology. His research interests include epidemiology, pathophysiologic mechanisms and management of hypertensive crisis, in addition to metabolic syndrome.

Contents

Preface

Cardiovascular diseases are the major cause of mortality in developed and developing countries. Hypertension is the most prevalent of all cardiovascular diseases, the major risk factor for cardio and cerebrovascular injury and the third cause of disability. It is likely to be involved in 50% of the deaths due to cardiovascular diseases. Genetic and environmental factors are involved in more than 90% of cases, characterizing essential hypertension. About 5 to 10% of hypertension cases are represented by cases of secondary arterial hypertension. In this situation, pheochromocytoma, a catechomine-secreting tumor that is located in the adrenal medulla (pheochromocytoma) or in the extra adrenal paraganglionic tissue (parangangliomа) presents prevalence varying from 0.01% to 0.10% of the hypertensive population, and an incidence of two to eight cases per million people per year.

When I received the invitation to be editor of a book on pheochromocytoma, a disease that represents small percentage of cases of secondary hypertension, I was worried with the development of the book and always wondered what would be the interest for the medical community. As the chapters were presented and developed by the authors, this worry has disappeared, because despite its rarity, pheochromocytoma presents a different clinical picture and several opportunities for clinical and basic research. Certainly, the level of the authors of this book also did make it an excellent topic to be discussed, in addition to chapters with new approaches about the clinical presentation and in the field of experimental research.

The book is divided into 6 sections covering the main aspects of clinical practice and other issues related to translational research. I hope readers enjoy this book and I expect it is a reference in the area.

Dr. Jose Fernando Vilela Martin, MD PhD,
Head of Internal Medicine Division,
Coordinator of Hypertension Clinic,
State Medical School of São José do Rio Preto (FAMERP),
Brazil

Part 1

Pathophysiology 1. Anatomo-Pathological Aspects

1

Macro and Microscopic Aspects

Fernando Candanedo-Gonzalez, Leslie Camacho-Rebollar
and Candelaria Cordova-Uscanga
*Department of Pathology, Oncology Hospital,
National Medical Center Century XXI,
Mexico City,
Mexico*

1. Introduction

In 1886, Fränkel first described pheochromocytoma at autopsy [1]. The term pheochromocytoma was coined by Poll in 1905 to describe the dusky (pheo) color (chromo) of the cut surface of the tumour when exposed to dichromate [2]. Not until 1926 did Mayo [3] at the Mayo Clinic and Roux [4] in Switzerland successfully remove these adrenal tumours. Interestingly, neither of these tumours was diagnosed preoperatively. Pheochromocytomas are rare catecholamine-producing neuroendocrine tumours arising from the chromaffin cells of the embryonic neural crest mainly of adrenal medulla or the extra-adrenal chromaffin tissue (paraganglia). Which synthesize, store, metabolize, and usually but not always secrete catecholamines.

1.1 Incidence

Population studies report an annual incidence of between 0.4 and 9.5 new cases per 100,000 adult persons each year [5,6,7], which constitute a curable form of hypertension in 0.1 to 1% of hypertension patients [8]. Of patients with pheochromocytoma discovered only at autopsy, 75% died suddenly from either myocardial infartion or a cerebrovascular catastrophe. Moreover, one third of the sudden deaths occurred during or immediately after unrelated minor operations [9,10]. Referrals for pheochromocytoma have been reported to be increasing, likely as a result of improved detection.

1.2 Clinical features

The majority of pheochromocytomas are sporadic in origin (80-90%) but may be associated with other diseases. Classically, pheochromocytomas has been termed a "10% tumour because roughly 10% of these tumours are malignant, multifocal, and bilateral, arise in extra-adrenal sites, and occur in children. However, recent evidence suggests the percentage of familial tumours is considerably higher [11].

1.3 Classic presentation

The classic triad of pheochromocytoma presentation is episodic headache, sweating, and palpitations. Manifestations of catecholamine excess form a wide spectrum of symptoms in these patients, the foremost being hypertension. Persistent hypertension is frequently considered part of the presentation. Also is typically found with a diverse set of symptoms, which may include anxiety, chest and abdominal pain, visual blurring, papilledema, nausea and vomiting, orthostatic hypotension, transitory electrocardiographic changes, and psychiatric disorders. As to be expected, these symptoms are not always present and certainly do not always constitute a diagnosis. Nonfunctioning pheochromocytomas are distinctly uncommon; nearly all patients with these tumours, at least in retrospect, demonstrate some characteristic symptom or sign, especially accentuated at the time of operative tumour manipulation. Diagnosis of pheochromocytoma includes detection of catecholamines in urine and plasma and radiological tests such as computed axial tomography, nuclear magnetic resonance imaging and metaiodobenzylguanidine scintigraphy. Laparoscopic techniques have become standard for treatment of tumours of the adrenal glands [12].

2. Pathology features

2.1 Macroscopy findings

Nearly 90% of pheochromocytomas are usually confined to the adrenal gland, and may appear encapsulated. In sporadic pheochromocytomas, even though lobulated, the tumour is actually a single neoplasm. In contrast, familial tumours are often bilateral and usually multicentric [13]. Pheochromocytomas are of variable size, ranging from 3 cm to 5 cm in diameter but can be more than 10 cm [14]. The weight may range from < 5g to over 3,500g, the average in patients with hypertension being 100g [15]. The cut surface is usually soft, yellowish white to reddish brown. The larger tumours often have areas of necrosis, hemorrhage, central degenerative change, cystic change and calcification. The normal gland can be seen in most cases but is sometimes attenuated (Fig. 1).

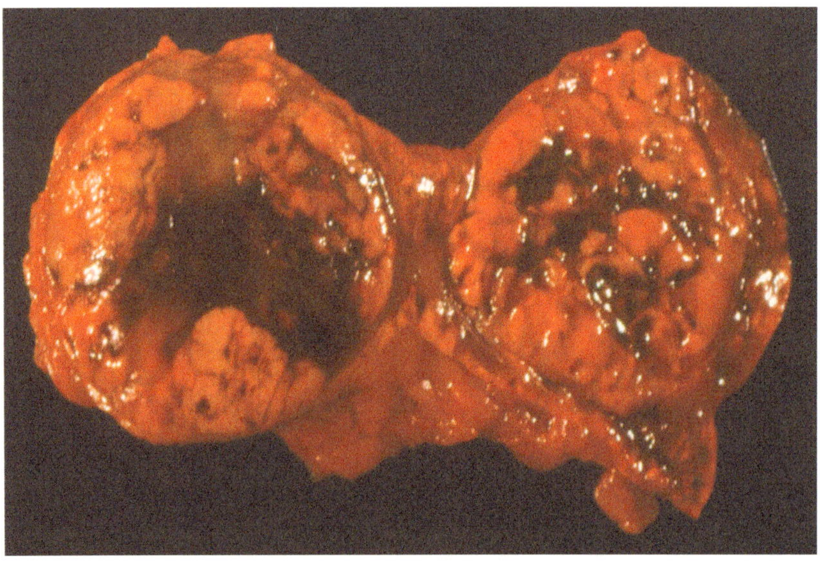

Fig. 1. Adrenal Pheochromocytoma. The round tumour extends torwards the adrenal cortex but is macroscopically well defined. Focal degenerative change and central hemorrhage is present. Attached adrenal remnant is also present.

The other 10 to 15% of cases are found in the neck, mediastinum and heart, or along the course of the sympathetic chain. The most frequent extra-adrenal site is the aortic bifurcation, the so-called organ of Zuckerkandl [16].

2.2 Histopathology

Microscopically, the tumour cells are characteristically arranged in well-defined nest ("Zellballen") or trabecular pattern bound by a delicate fibrovascular stroma, or a mixture of the two (Fig. 2A). Diffuse or solid architecture can also be seen. A true capsule does not usually separate the tumour from the adjacent adrenal but a pseudocapsule may be present, or the tumour may extend to the adrenal capsule. The border with the adjacent cortex may be irregular, with intermingling of tumour cells with cortical cells.

The tumour cells vary considerably in size and shape and have a finely granular basophilic or amphophilic cytoplasm. The nuclei are usually round or oval with prominent nucleoli and may contain inclusion-like structure resulting from deep cytoplasmic invaginations. Cellular and nuclear pleomorphism is sometimes prominent (Fig. 2B) [17]. Spindle cells are present in about 2% of cases, usually as a minor component. Haemorrhage and haemosiderin deposits are common. Mitotic figures are rare, with an average of one per 30 high power fields reported in clinically benign lesions [18].

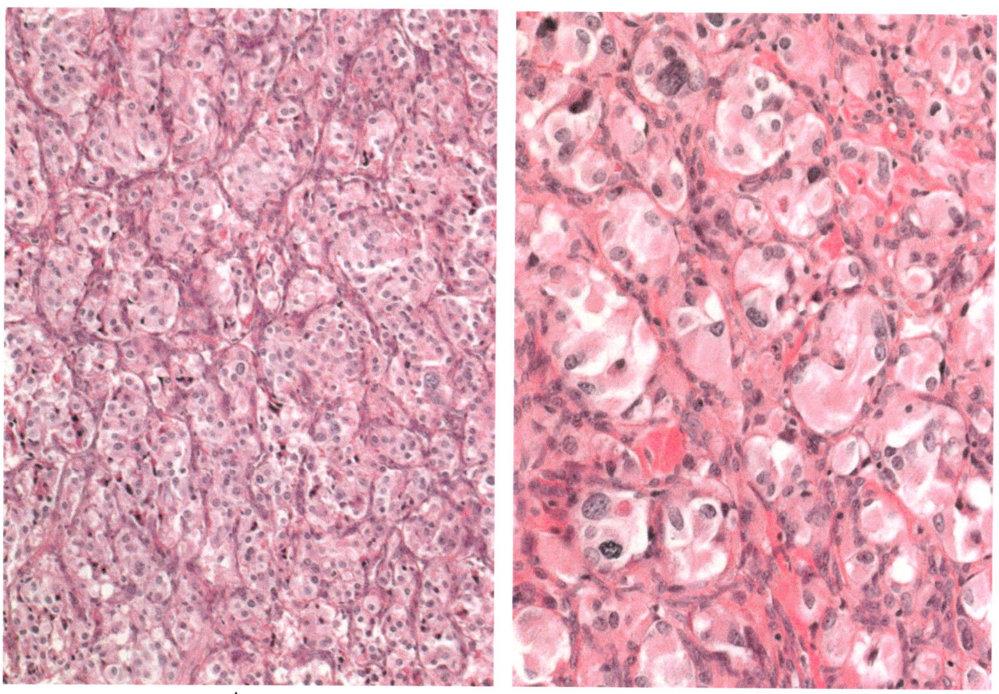

A B

Fig. 2. Benign pheochromocytoma. **A)** Well-defined nest of cuboidal cells are separated by highly vascularized fibrous septa ("zellballen"). A granular, basophilic cytoplasm is usually identified surrounding slightly irregular nuclei; **B)** nuclear pleomorphisms are sometimes prominent.

2.3 Immunohistochemistry

Specific diagnosis is usually based on morphology and confirmed by immunohistochemistry. Pheochromocytomas are positive for chromogranin A. Other neural markers such as synaptophysin have been reported to be variably positive in cortical tumours. The absence of positivity for epithelial membrane antigen helps distinguish pheochromocytoma from renal cell carcinoma. Immunostaining for S100 protein will demonstrate sustentacular cells [19] which are usually arranged around the periphery of the cell nests where there is an alveolar arrangement (Fig. 3).

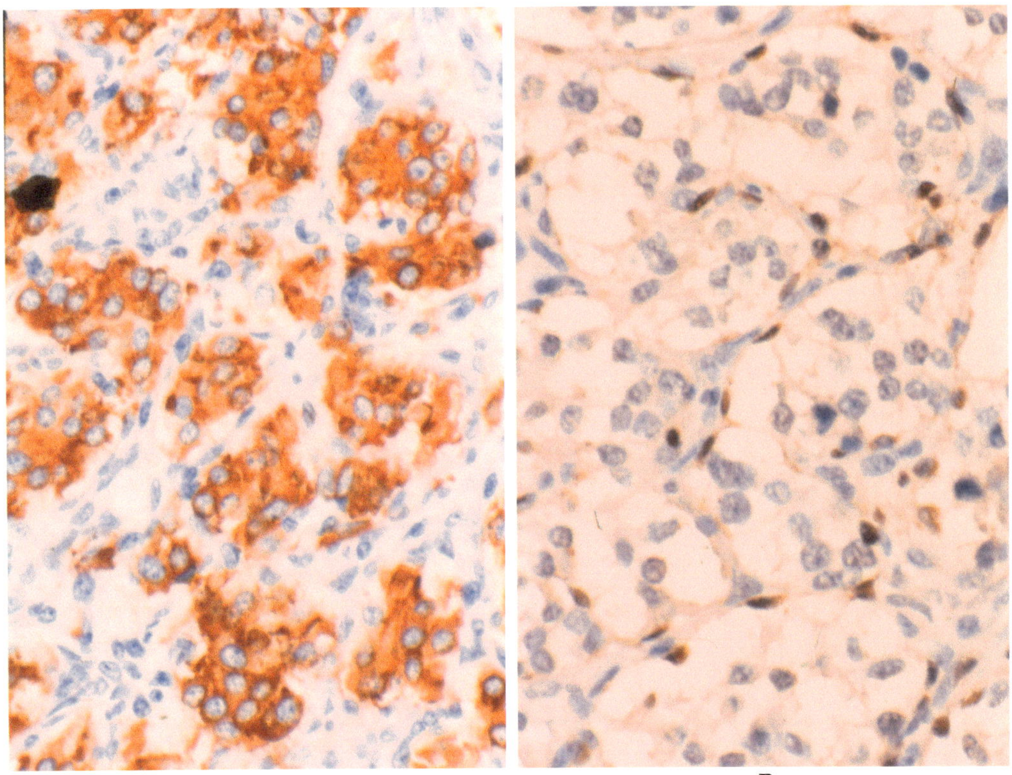

A B

Fig. 3. Immunohistochemical staining. **A)** Positive cytoplasmic immunostain for chromogranin in the pheochromocytoma; **B)** Immunostain for S-100 protein shows intense dark staining of elongated nuclei of sustentacular cells. These are usually located near vascular channels.

3. Familial pheochromocytoma

Pheochromocytomas are considered to be unique neuroendocrine tumours since they can occur as part of several familial tumour syndromes. It is now recognized that the frequency of germline mutations in apparently sporadic presentations is as high as 15%–24% [11,20]. However, the genetic basis of the majority of sporadic pheochromocytomas remains largely uncharacterized.

Familial pheochromocytomas are often multifocal or bilateral and generally present at an earlier age than sporadic pheochromocytoma. Germline mutations in six genes have been associated with familial pheochromocytoma, namely, the von Hippel-Lindau gene (*VHL*), which causes von Hippel-Lindau (VHL) syndrome, the *RET* gene, leading to multiple endocrine neoplasia type 2 (MEN 2), the neurofibromatosis type 1 gene (*NF1*), associated with neurofibromatosis type 1 (NF1) disease, and the genes encoding subunits B and D (and also rarely C) of mitochondrial succinate dehydrogenase (*SDHB, SDHD*, and *SDHC*), which are associated with familial paraganglioma/PPC. The recent description of mutations of the succinate dehydrogenase gene (*SDH*) has demonstrated a much stronger hereditary component than formerly thought. Currently, up to 24% of pheochromocytomas may have a genetic predisposition [11,20].
The genetic susceptibility of malignant and benign pheochromocytomas is similar. However, advances in molecular genetics continue to underscore the importance of hereditary factors in the development of pheochromocytoma and propensity to malignancy. Malignant tumours have been reported in patients with germline mutations of *RET, VHL, NF1* and the *SDH* genes [21,22]. On the other hand, malignant pheochromocytomas in the setting of MEN 2 occur less frequently than sporadic tumours [23,24,25,26]. Which suggesting certain groups are predisposed to malignant disease. For example, patients with *SDHB* mutations are more likely to develop malignant disease and nondiploid tumours have also been found to be associated with malignancy. Gene expression and protein profiling are beginning to identify the genetic characteristics of malignant pheochromocytoma. However, the genetic changes that induce malignant disease remain unclear.

4. Malignant disease

Most pheochromocytomas are benign and curable by surgical resection, but some are clinically malignant [27]. The pathologist cannot determine whether a tumour is benign or malignant based on histological features alone. Although extensive invasion of adjacent tissues can be considered an indicator of malignant potential, local invasiveness and malignant disease are not necessarily associated. Currently, there are no prognostic tests that can reliably predict which patients are at risk of developing metastatic disease. The World Health Organization tumour definition of a malignant pheochromocytoma is the presence of metastases, at site distant where chromaffin cells do not normally exist [28]. Metastases occur most frequently to bone, liver, lungs and regional lymph nodes, and can appear as many as 20 years after initial presentation, which implies that life-long follow-up of patients (Fig. 4) [29].
Some studies have suggested that the presence of necrosis, vascular invasion, extensive local invasion, and high rate of mitotic figures may indicate a malignant behavior in pheochromocytoma. Indeed, a recent study by Thompson used clinical features, histologic findings, and immunophenotypic studies to indentify parameters that may help distinguish benign from malignant pheochromocytoma of the Adrenal Gland Scaled Score (PASS) as a scoring system to differentiate benign from malignant pheochromocytomas. PASS is weighted for 12 specific histologic features that are more frequently identified in malignant pheochromocytomas. Factors such as tumour necrosis, high mitotic rate, tumour cell spindling, and vascular invasion are included in this scoring system (Fig. 5). Thompson found that tumours with ≥4 were biologically more aggressive than tumours with a PASS <4, which behaved in a benign fashion (Table 1) [30].

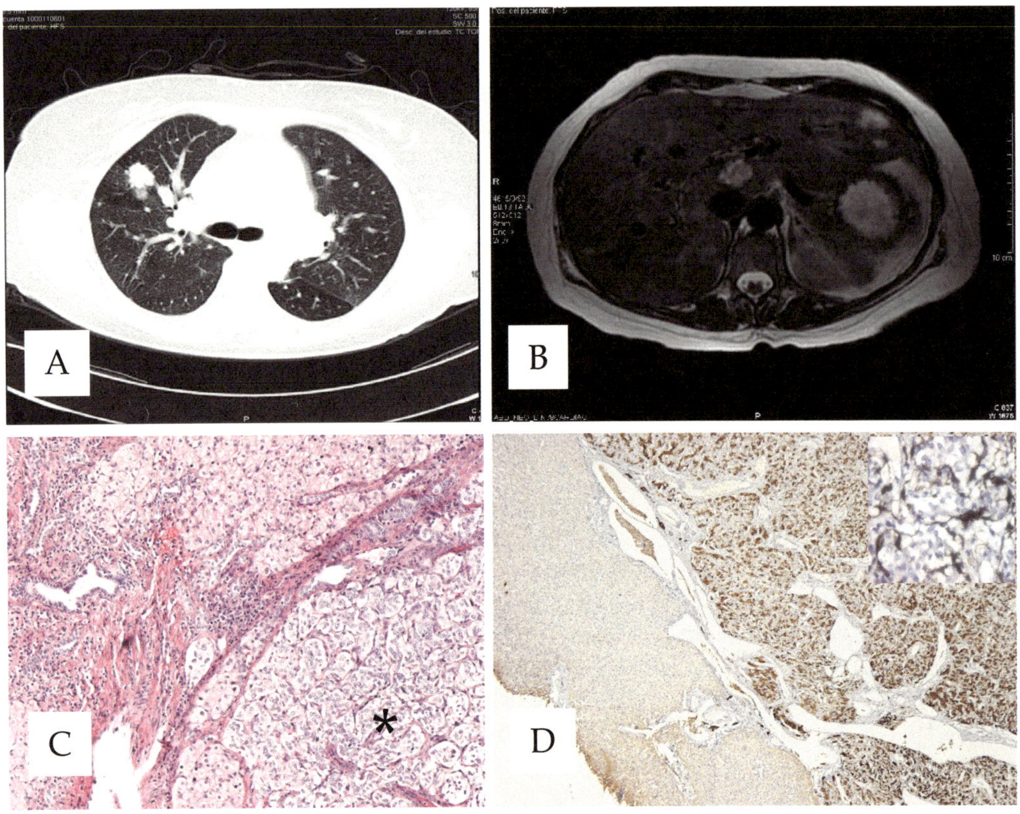

Fig. 4. Malignant pheochromocytoma. **A** and **B)** Multiple liver and lungs metastatic lesions were shown by computed tomography; **C)** Transition from the metastatic pheochromocytoma component (*) to the liver within the same section; **D)** By immunohistochemical was confirmed the presence of a metastatic pheochromocytoma with the characteristic chromogranin immunoreactivity in the pheochromocytos and the S-100 protein immunoreactivity of the sustentacular cells which contrasted with negative liver tissue.

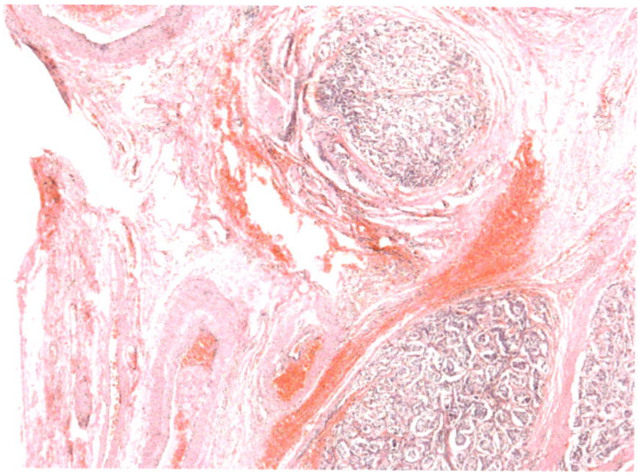

A

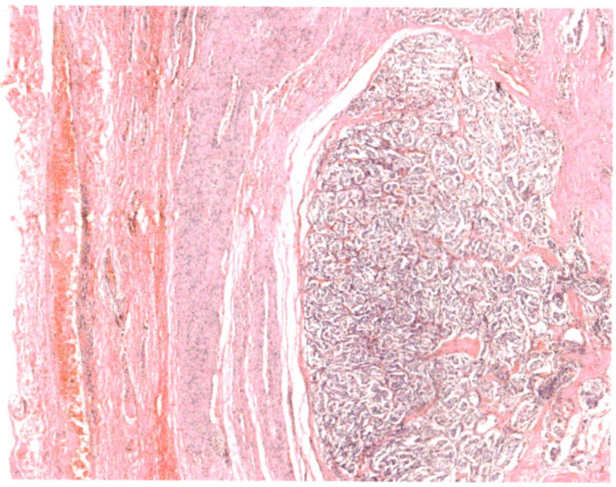

B

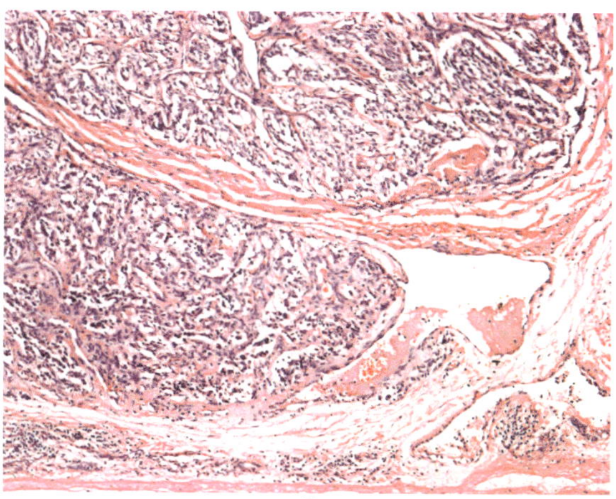

C

Fig. 5. Invasive malignant pheochromocytoma. **A)** A thick fibrous capsule is transgressed by the neoplastic cells with extension into surrounding addipose connective tissue in malignant pheochromocytoma; **B)** Extension into a vascular spaces is noted in a malignant pheochromocytoma.

Microscopic feature	Score
Extension into peri-adrenal adipose tissue	2
Presence of large nests or diffuse growth (>10% of tumour volume)†	2
Central tumour necrosis (in the middle of large nests or confluent necrosis)	2
High cellularity	2
Tumour cell spindling even when focal	2
Cellular monotony	2
Mitotic figures >3/10 high-power field	2
Atypical mitotic figures	2
Vascular invasion*	1
Capsular invasion	1
Profound nuclear pleomorphism	1
Nuclear hyperchromasia	1
Total	20

*Defined by direct extension into vessel lumen, intravascular attached tumour thrombi, and/ or tumour nests convered by endothelium identified in a capsular or extracapsular vessel.
†Defined as 3-4 times the size of a zellballen or the normal size of the medullary paraganglia nest.

Table 1. Pheochromocytoma of the Adrenal Gland Scoring Scale (PASS) [30].

Additional markers that might be useful prognostic indicators in the pathological assessment of these tumours are sought. However, some studies with markers for important events in the cell cycle showed that less $p21/^{WAF1}$ expression and aneuploidy correlated with malignant pheochromocytomas [31,32,33].

4.1 Prognosis and predictive factors

The rarity of this tumours and the resulting fragmented nature of studies, typically involving small numbers of patients, represent limiting factors to the development of effective treatments and diagnostic or prognostic markers for malignant disease. The prognosis for patients with benign pheochromocytoma is primarily dependent upon a successful surgical resection and extend of preoperative complications related to hypertension. The usual prognosis of malignant pheochromocytoma is poor, with a 45-55% 5-year survival [30,34,35,36,37,38]. However, some patients may have indolent disease, with life expectancy of more than 20 years [39]. Until further studies identify precise biological markers that can accurately predict the clinical behaviour of catecholamine-secreting tumours, it may be advisable for all pheochromocytoma patients to undergo lifelong hormonal monitoring and imaging studies to detect recurrence and metastases [40].

5. Composite pheochromocytoma

Ordinary pheochromocytoma is composed of polygonal to spindled cells arranged in an alveolar, trabecular, or solid pattern, often with a typical Zellballen appearance. Composite pheochromocytomas account for only 3% of both adrenal and extra-adrenal pheochromocytomas and can be associated with MEN 2A and phakomatoses [41,42]. Composite pheochromocytoma is a rare tumour composed of typical pheochromocytoma and other components, most often neuroblastoma [43], ganglioneuroblastoma, or ganglioneuroma in adult cases, and pediatric were very rare. Rare cases have displayed pheochromocytoma with other coexisting neural or neural crest-derived tumours such as malignant peripheral nerve sheath tumour. Little is known about the biologic potential, outcome, or molecular genetic profile.

Because composite pheochromocytoma clinically resembles a typical pheochromocytoma, diagnosis is frequently made by the pathologist. The median age is 16 yr (9 to 24 yr) [43]. The pathologic diagnosis of composite pheochromocytomas creates a clinical dilemma because it is not known whether the neuroblastic component results in therapeutic and prognostic implications different from those in ordinary pheochromocytoma. Neuroblastoma is the most immature of the neuroblastic tumours; the others are ganglioneuroblastoma and ganglioglioma (Table 2). These tumours are differentiated based on the amount of schwannian stroma and the presence or absence of ganglion cell differentiation. This dual phenotype is supported by light microscopy and corroborated by immunohistochemistry and ultrastructural findings. Prognosis of coexistence with pheochromocytoma and ganglioneuroblastoma or neuroblastoma is variable.

Coexistence with	No. of cases	%
Ganglioneuroma	41	70
Ganglioneuroblastoma	7	11
Neuroblastoma	4	9
Schwannoma	4	7
Neuroendocrine carcinoma	1	2
Total	57	100

Table 2. Cases of composite pheochromocytoma of adrenal gland [43].

6. New insights on pheochromocytoma

The molecular events involved in the malignant transformation of pheochromocytoma are poorly understood. There are also no reliable and uniformly accepted histopathologic criteria to distinguish benign from malignant pheochromocytoma. Unsupervised cluster analysis showed 3 main clusters of tumors that did not have complete concordance with the clinical and pathologic groupings of pheochromocytomas. Supervised cluster analysis showed almost completely separate clustering between benign and malignant tumours. The differentially expressed genes with known function belonged to 8 biologic process categories; signal transduction, transcription, protein transport, protein synthesis, smooth muscle contraction, ion transport, chemotaxis, and electron transport. Gene set enrichment analysis revealed significant correlation between the microarray profiles of malignant pheochromocytomas and several known molecular pathways associated with carcinogenesis and dedifferentiation. Ten differentially expressed genes had high diagnostic accuracy, and 5 of these genes (CFC1, FAM62B, HOMER1, LRRN3, TBX3, ADAMTS) in combination distinguishing benign versus malignant tumours. Differentially expressed genes between benign and malignant pheochromocytomas distinguish between these tumours with high diagnostic accuracy. These findings provide new insight into the genes and molecular pathways that may be involved in malignant pheochromocytomas [44].

7. Future directions

Much attention has recently been devoted to pheochromocytoma as the understanding of this disease continues to improve. If it becomes widely available, it would greatly aid in the staging and management of malignant disease. Continually improving detection methods, especially screening of high-risk populations, will only contribute to the treatment and knowledge of these conditions in the future. It has become clear that many apparently sporadic pheochromocytomas have a genetic component. Not only has there been a great deal of attention directed toward the hereditary components, but better predictive molecular factors have been identified for malignant pheochromocytoma, which could lead to more effective genetic testing. In addition, microarray studies have identified a set of genes preferentially expressed in malignant pheochromocytoma. The combination of an identifiable hereditary component along with an understanding of the genetic and molecular defects in sporadic pheochromocytoma makes this a promising model and approach for insights into other cancers. The future is wide open for improvements in the understanding and treatment of this disease.

8. References

[1] Fränkel F. Ein fall von doppelseitigen vollig latent verlaufen nebennier entumor und gleichseitiger nephritis mit veranderungen am circulation sappart und retinitis. Virchow Arch [A] 1886;103:244.

[2] Poll H. Die vergleichende Entwicklung der nebennierensysteme. In: Hertwig O, ed. Handbuch der Entwicklungsgeschichte des Menschen und der Wirbeltiere. Jena: Gustave Fishcer, 1905:443-448.

[3] Mayo CH. Paroxystmal hypertension with tumor of retroperitoneal nerve. JAMA 1927;89:1047.

[4] Roux C. Thesis Lausanne. Cited by Welbourne RB. Early surgical history of pheochromocytoma. Br J Surg 1987;74:594.

[5] De Graeff J, Horak BJV. The incidence of phaeochromocytoma in the Netherlands. Acta Med Scand 1964;176:583-593.

[6] Beard CM, Sheps SG, Kurland LT, Carney JA, Lie JT. Ocurrence of pheochromocytoma in Rochester, Minnesota, 1950 through 1979. Mayo Clin Proc 1983;58:802-804.

[7] Sheps SG, Jiang NS, Klee GG. Diagnostic evaluation of pheochromocytoma. Endocrinol Metab Clin North Am 1988;17:397-414.

[8] Samaan NA, Hickey RC, Shutts PE. Diagnosis, localization, and management of pheochromocytoma: Pitfalls and follow-up in 41 patients. Cancer 1988;62:2451-2460.

[9] Graham JB. Phaeochromocytoma and hypertension; an analysis of 207 cases. Int Abstr Surg 1951;92:105-121.

[10] Sutton MG, Sheps SG, Lie JT. Prevalence of clinically unsuspected pheochromocytoma: review of a 50-year autopsy series. Mayo Clin Proc 1981;56:354-360.

[11] Neumann HP, Bausch B, McWhinney SR, Bender BU, Gimm O, Franke G, Schipper J, Klisch J, Altehoefer C, Zerres K, Januszewicz A, Eng C, Smith WM, Munk R, Manz T, Glaesker S, Apel TW, Treier M, Reineke M, Walz MK, Hoang-Vu C, Brauckhoff M, Klein-Franke A, Klose P, Schmidt H, Maier-Woelfle M, Peczkowska M, Szmigielski C. Germ-line mutations in nonsyndromic pheochromocytoma. N Engl J Med 2002;346:1459-1466.

[12] Gil-Cárdenas A, Cordón C, Gamino R, Rull JA, Gómez-Pérez F, Pantoja JP, Herrera MF. Laparoscopic adrenalectomy: lessons learned from and initial series of 100 patients. Surg Endosc 2008;22:991-994.
[13] Webb TA, Sheps SG, Carney JA. Differences between sporadic pheochromocytoma and pheochromocytoma in multiple endocrine neoplasia type 2. Am J Surg Pathol 1980;4:121-126.
[14] Page DL, DeLellis RA, Hough AJJ. Tumors of the Adrenal. 2nd ed. Armed Forces Institute of Pathology: Washington, D.C.
[15] ReMine WH, Chong GC, van Heerden JA, Sheps SG, Harrison EGJr. Current management of pheochromocytoma. Ann Surg 1974;179:740-748.
[16] van Heerden JA, Sheps SG, Hamberger B, Sheedy PF 2nd, Poston JG, ReMine WH. Pheochromocytoma: Current status and changing trends. Surgery 1982;91:367-373.
[17] DeLellis RA, Suchow E, Wolfe HJ. Ultrastructure of nuclear "inclusions" in pheochromocytoma and paraganglioma. Hum Pathol 1980;11:205-207.
[18] Linnoila RI, Keiser HR, Steinberg SM, Lack EE. Histopathology of benign versus malignant sympathoadrenal paragangliomas: clinicopathologic study of 120 cases including unusual histologic features. Hum Pathol 1990;21:1168-1180.
[19] Lloyd RV, Blaivas M, Wilson BS. Distribution of chromogranin and S100 protein in normal and abnormal adrenal medullary tissues. Arch Pathol Lab Med 1985;109:633-635.
[20] Bryant J, Farmer J, Kessler LJ, Townsend RR, Nathanson KL. Pheochromocytoma: the expanding genetic differential diagnosis. J Nat Cancer Ints 2003;1196-1204.
[21] Koch CA, Vortmeyer AO, Huang SC, Alesci S, Zhuang Z, Pacak K. Genetic aspects of pheochromocytoma. Endocr Regul 2001;35:43-52.
[22] Neumann HP, Berger DP, Sigmund G, Blum U, Schmidt D, Parmer RJ, Volk B, Kriste G. Pheochromocytomas, multiple endocrine neoplasia type 2, and von Hippel-Lindau disease. N Engl J Med 1993;329:1531-1538.
[23] Casanova S, Rosenberg-Bourgin M, Farkas D, Calmettes C, Feingold N, Heshmati HM, Cohen R, Conte-Devolx B, Guillausseau PJ, Houdent C, Bigogne JC, Boiteau V, Caron J, Modigliani E. Phaeochromocytoma in multiple endocrine neoplasia type 2 A: survey of 100 cases. Clin Endocrinol (Oxf) 1993;38:531-537.
[24] Medeiros LJ, Wolf BC, Balogh K, Federman M. Adrenal pheochromocytoma: a clinicopathologic review of 60 cases. Hum Pathol 1985;16:580-589.
[25] Modigliani E, Vasen HM, Raue K, Dralle H, Frilling A, Gheri RG, Brandi ML, Limbert E, Niederle B, Forgas L, Rosenberg-Bourgin M, Calmettes C. Pheochromocytoma in multiple endocrine neoplasia type 2: European study. The Euromen Study Group. J Intern Med 1995;238:363-367.
[26] Scopsi L, Catellani MR, Gullo M, Cusumato F, Camerini E, Pasini B, Orefice S. Malignant pheochromocytoma in multiple endocrine neoplasia type 2B syndrome. Case report and review of the literature. Tumori 1996;82:480-484.
[27] Lehnert H, Mundschenk J, Hahn K. Malignant pheochromocytoma. Front Horm Res 2004;31:155-162.
[28] DeLellis RA, Lloyd RV, Heitz PU, Eng C. Eds 2004. Tumours of Endocrine Organs. IARC Press. Lyon.
[29] Strong VE, Kennedy T, Al-Ahmadie H, Tang L, Coleman J, Fong Y, Brennan M, Ghossein RA. Prognostic indicators of malignancy in adrenal pheochromocytomas:

clinical, histopathologic, and cell cycle/apoptosis gene expression analysis. Surgery 2008;143:759-768.
[30] Thompson LDR. Pheochromocytoma of the Adrenal Gland Scaled Score (PASS) to separate benign from malignant neoplasms. A clinicopathologic and immunophenotypic study of 100 cases. Am J Surg Pathol 2002;26:551-566.
[31] Candanedo-Gonzalez F, Barraza IB, Cerbulo VA, Saqui SM, Gamboa DA. Aneuplody and low p21/WAF1 expression in malignant paragangliomas. Virchow Archiv 2005;447:430.
[32] Nativ O, Grant CS, Sheps SG, O'Fallon JR, Farrow GM, van Heerden JA, Lieber MM. The clinical significance of nuclear DNA ploidy pattern in 184 patients with pheochromocytoma. Cancer 1992;69:2683-2687.
[33] Carisen E, Abdullan Z, Kazmi SM, Kousparos G. Pheochromocytomas, PASS, and immunohistochemistry. Horm Metab Res 2009;41: 715-719.
[34] Modlin IM, Farndon JR, Shepherd A, Johnston ID, Kennedy TL, Montgomery DA, Welbourn RB. Phaeochromocytomas in 72 patients: clinical and diagnostic features, treatment and long term results. Br J Surg 1979;66:456-465.
[35] Pommier RF, Vetto JT, Bilingsly K, Woltering EA, Brennan MF. Comparison of adrenal and extra-adrenal pheochromocytomas. Surgery 1993;114:1160-1165.
[36] Scott HWJr, Halter SA. Oncologic aspects of pheochromocytoma: importance of follow-up. Surgery 1984:96:1061-1066.
[37] Reynolds V, Green N, Page D, Oates JA, Robertson D, Roberts S. Clinical experience with malignant pheochromocytomas. Surg Gynecol Obstet 1982;154:801-818.
[38] Shapiro B, Sisson JC, Lloyd R, Nakajo M, Satterlee W, Beierwaltes WH. Malignant phaeochromocytoma: clinical, biochemical and scintigraphic characterization. Clin Endocrinol (Oxf) 1984;20:189-203.
[39] Young AL, Baysal BE, Deb A, Young WF Jr. Familial malignant catecholamine-secreting parganglioma with prolonged survival associated with mutation in the succinate dehydrogenase B gene. J Clin Endocrinol Metab 2002;87:4101-4105.
[40] Tang SH, Chen A, Lee CT, Yu DS, Chang SY, Sun GH. Remote recurrence of malignant pheochromocytoma 14 years after primary operation. J Urol 2003;169:269.
[41] Jansson S, Dahlstrom A, Hansson G, Tisell LE, Ahlman H. Concomitant occurrence of an adrenal ganglioneuroma and a contralateral pheochromocytoma in a patient with von Recklinghausen's neurofibromatosis. An immunocytochemical study. Cancer 1989;63:324-329.
[42] Tischler AS. Divergent differentiation in neuroendocrine tumors of the adrenal gland. Semin Diagn Pathol 2000;17:120-126.
[43] Candanedo Gonzalez F, Alvarado Cabrero I, Gamboa Dominguez A, Cerbulo Vazquez A, Lopez Romero R, Bornstein Quevedo L, Salcedo Vargas M. Sporadic type composite pheochromocytoma with neuroblastoma: clinicomorphologic, DNA content, and ret gene analysis. Endocrine Pathol 2001;12:343-350.
[44] Suh I, Shribru D, Eisenhofer G, Pacak K, Duh QY, Crack OH, Kebebew E. Candidate genes associated with malignant pheochromocytomas by genome-wide expression profiling. Ann Surg 2009;983-990.

2

Phaechromocytoma with Histopathologic Aspects

Servet Guresci, Derun Taner Ertugrul and Gulcin Guler Simsek
Kecioren Training and Research Hospital
Turkey

1. Introduction

Phaeochromocytoma is a term used for catecholamine secreting tumors that arise from chromaffin cells of sympathetic paraganglia. The new World Health Organisation (WHO) classification of endocrine tumors has recommended to reserve the term phaeochromocytoma for intraadrenal tumors only and the others are defined as sympathetic or parasympathetic paragangliomas, further categorised by site. Although it was the first adrenal tumor to be recognised, the term phaeochromocytoma was introduced many years later by Pick in 1912. The name is based on the fact that the tumors get dark brown after exposure to potassium dichromate because of chromaffin reaction.

2. The usual adrenal medulla

2.1 Anatomy

The human adrenal glands are located in retroperitoneum superomedial to kidneys. They are composite endocrine organs made up of cortex and medulla which have different embriyonic origin, function and histology. On fresh or formalin fixated cut surface the two portions, a relatively thick outer yellow cortex and inner, pearly gray medulla, is readily visible. The medulla is mainly situated in head and partly body of the organ . It may variably extend to tail and focally to alae. It's weight comprises about 8%-10% of the total. Medulla is of neuroectodermal origin and secretes and stores catecholamines, especially epinephrine.

2.2 Histology

On histological examination the cortex-medulla junction is sharp with no intervening connective tissue but the border is irregular. The medulla is mainly composed of chromaffin cells (phaeochromocytes, medullary cells) that are arranged in tight clusters and trabeculae seperated by a reticular fiber network. Embriyologically, they are modified sympathetic postganglionic neurons which have lost their axons. They are all innervated by cholinergic endings of preganglionic symptathetic neurons. There are sustentacular cells at the periphery of clusters which can only be demonstrated by immunostaining for S-100 protein. The chromaffin cells are polygonal to columnar and larger than cortical cells. They have basophilic cytoplasm which have fine secretory granules and/or vacuoles. These granules contain catecholamines and derivates of tyrosine which transform to colored polymers by

oxidizing agents such as potassium dichromate and ferric chloride. This staining is called chromaffin reaction which is replaced by formaldehyde methods for detection of catecholamins because of its relatively low sensitivity.
Among chromaffin cells are randomly scattered individual or group of parasympathetic ganglion cells that are often associated with a nerve. Small clusters of cortical cells are also a usual component of the medulla. Small groups of lymphocytes and plasma cells may be seen within the medulla but their significance is unknown.

2.3 Ultrastructure

Ultrastructural examinations have shown that epinephrine and norepinephrine are secreted by two different types of cells. Epinephrine secreting cells have smaller, moderately electron-dense granules that are closely applied to their limiting membranes. Norepinephrine secreting cells' granules are larger, more electron-dense and have an electron-lucent layer beneath the surrounding membrane forming a halo. The nuclei are usually larger than cortical cells and have finely or coarsely clumped chromatin. Most nuclei are spheroidal and show slight pleomorphism.

3. The paraganglia

Sympathetic paraganglia (SP) are distributed along paraaxial regions of the trunk along the prevertebral and paravertebral sympathetic chains and in connective tissue in the walls of pelvic organs. However parasympathetic paraganglia (PSP) are found along cranial and thoracic branches of the glossopharyngeal and vagus nerves. Among SP the organ of Zuckerkandl is characteristic, located at the origin of the inferior mesenteric artery, because of being the only macroscopic extraadrenal paraganglia. Similarly PSP are highly variable in number and location and don't have specific names except from carotid bodies which are located between the carotid arteries just above the carotid bifurcation. Apart from different clinical standpoint SP and PSP are similar at cellular level.

4. Histopathology of phaeochromocytoma

Sporadic phaeochromocytomas make up of about 50% of all phaeochromocytomas and are usually unilateral and unicentric while more than 50% of familial forms are bilateral and coexist with extraadrenal sympathetic and parasympathetic paragangliomas. Patients with MEN type 2, VHL or NF type 1 are known to have an increased risk for pheochromocytoma.

4.1 Macroscopic examination

Gross examination highligts a tumor 3-5 cm in diameter which can be more than 10 cm. Tumor weight may range from a few grams to over 3500g, with an average of 100 g in hypertension patients. The cut surface is solid, gray-white, light tan or dusky red and darkens on exposure to air (Figure 1). Hemorrhage, central degeneration, necrosis, cytic change and calcification is not uncommon. The adrenal gland can usually be seen compressed or incorporated within the tumor. An adrenal gland containing phaeochromocytoma should be carefully dissected since diffuse and nodular hyperplasia can be found suggestive of a familial form.

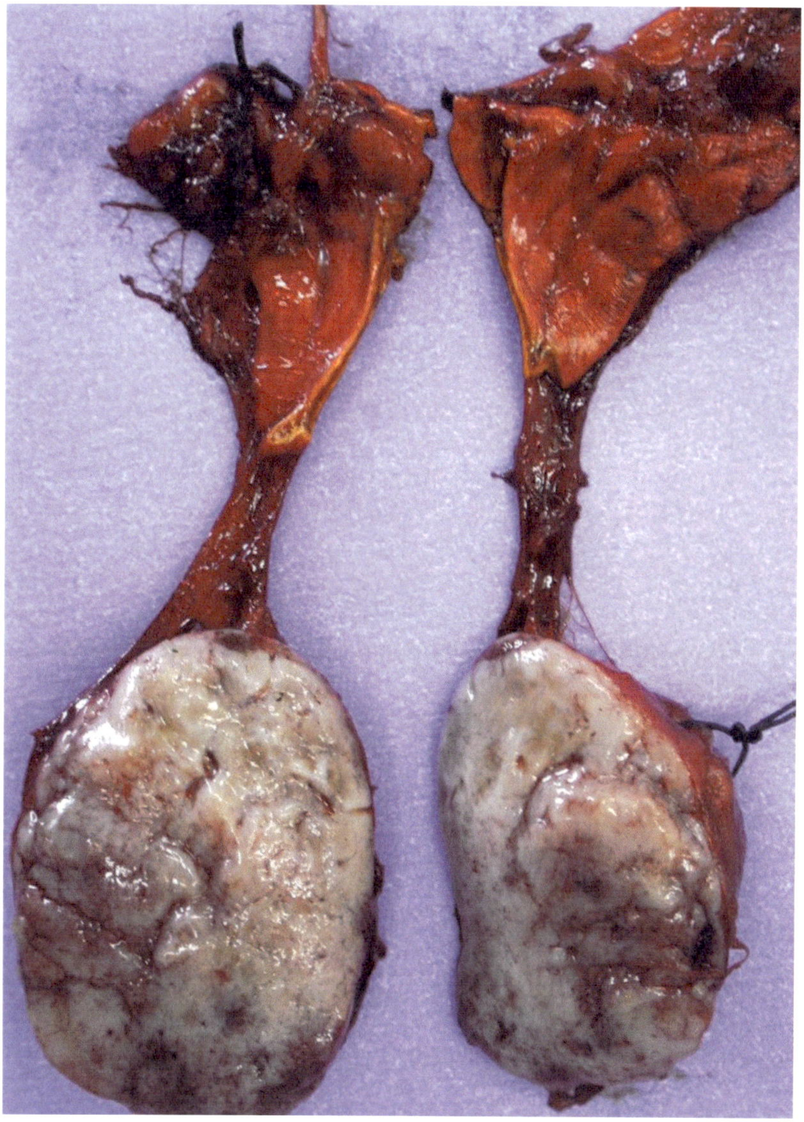

Fig. 1. Extra-adrenal paraganglioma with a nodular, tan cut surface. Adrenal gland can be encountered in orange above the tumor (by courtesy of Prof. Dr. Filiz Ozyilmaz).

4.2 Microscopic examination

Microscopically, similar to usual corticomedullary border,cortex-tumor border is irregular and there's a pseudocapsule rather than a true capsule. The most common histologic pattern is alveolar (Zellballen) and trabecular or a mixture of the two, bound by a delicate fibrovascular stroma (Figure 2). Diffuse or solid pattern can also be encountered. Tumor cells resemble usual chromaffin cells but are slightly larger. Sometimes nuclear and cellular pleomorphism is pronounced. Nuclear pseudoinclusions can be seen resulting from deep cytoplasmic invaginations. Occasional mitotic figures are present but they don't exceed 1/30 hpf. Intracytoplasmic hyaline globules are common. Their presence may aid to differentiate phaeochromocytoma from adrenal cortical neoplasms. Interstitial amyloid deposition and small amounts of melanin pigment representing neuromelanin may be present . Hemorrhage and hemosiderin deposits are common and scattered ganglion cells can be encountered. Sometimes tumor cells may undergo lipid degeneration and this may lead to confusion with cortical tumors. Exceptionally, the cells of phaeochromocytoma may contain a large number of mitochondria which give the cells oncocytic appearance. Spindle shaped sustentacular cells form a second cell component of phaeochromocytoma forming a peripheral rim around Zellballen, similar to usual adrenal medulla. These cells have been encountered more frequently in phaeochromocytomas associated with MEN and benign forms.

Histopathologic diagnosis of phaeochromocytoma is based on morphology but immunohistochemical techniques are usually used to confirm the diagnosis. Immunopositivity for neuron spesific enolase, chromogranin-A and synaptophysin is characteristic.

Extra-adrenal SP are mostly solitary in adults and histologically resemble adrenal counterpart. Dispersed along the paravertebral sympathetic chain, they are most common in the superior (45%) followed by inferior (30%) paraaortic region. Urinary bladder, intrathoracic and cervical paragangliomas can occasionally be seen. More than 25% of these tumors are functional and usually secrete norepinephrine. Approximately 50% of extraadrenal tumors are malignant giving rise to metastases.

PSP seldomly produce cathecolamine excess. Carotid body and jugulotympanic tumors are more common than aortic and vagal lesions. Carotid body tumors are more commonly bilateral in familial cases . Also people living at high altitude is ten times at a higher risk for paraganglioma because of hyperplastic response to hypoxic stimulus.

4.2.1 Malignant phaeochromocytoma

Malignant phaeochromocytomas comprise up to 10% of all phaeochromocytomas. WHO 2004 classification of endocrine tumors defines malignant phaeochromocytoma only when there is metastasis to sites where paraganglial tissue is not otherwise found. As a matter of fact there's no reliable histological criteria for classifiying phaeochromocytoma as malignant at present, therefore no lesion can be definetly predicted as benign. There are new approaches to find significant histologic criteria for defining phaeochromocytoma malignant. Large nests of tumor cells, necrosis, high cellularity, cellular monotony, nuclear hyperchromasia, macronucleoli, vascular or capsular invasion, increased mitotic figures and high Ki-67 proliferation index, extension of tumor into adjacent fat, catecholamine phenotype and absence of hyaline globules are all shown to be correlated with malignant behaviour in scoring studies in both phaeochromocytomas and extraadrenal sympathetic

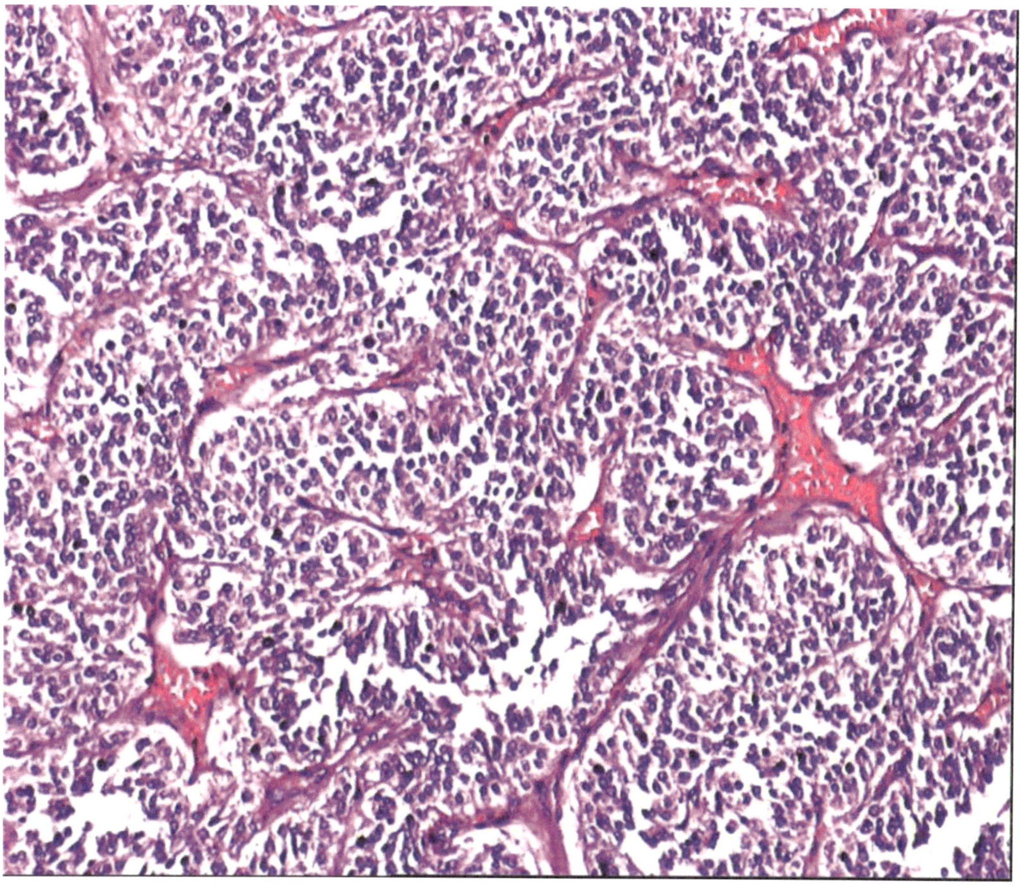

Fig. 2. Typical Zellballen pattern of phaeochromocytoma (HEx200) (by courtesy of Prof. Dr. Filiz Ozyilmaz).

paragangliomas. Unfortunately none of these criteria give exact discrimination thus histological gold standard is still not possessed.

4.2.2 Composite phaeochromocytoma

Composite phaeochromocytoma or paraganglioma refers to histological combination of phaeochromocytoma and paraganglioma with features of ganglioneuroma, ganglioneuroblastoma, neuroblastoma or peripheral nerve sheath tumour. There are fewer than 40 cases in the literature. The tumour was combined with ganglioneuroma in 80%, and with ganglioneuroma in 20% of all reported cases. They are usually seen in adults and symptoms are similar to typical phaeochromocytoma as with genetic abnormalities. About 90% occur in adrenal gland and the remainder in the urinary bladder. Altough ordinary phaeochromocytomas can contain scattered neuron-like or ganglion cells the histopathological diagnosis of composite tumour requires both different architecture and cell population. Present evidences show that the origin of neurons in these tumours is preexisting chromaffin or paraganglioma cells. Cell culture studies favor that both normal and neoplastic human phaeochromocytoma cells can undergo neuronal differentiaton.

4.2.3 Adrenal medullary hyperplasia

Lastly, diffuse or nodular adrenal medullary hyperplasia may cause exess amount of cathecolamine secretion and may lead to clinical phaeochromocytoma.

5. Conclusion

It is easy to define usual phaeochromocytoma histopathologically but diagnosing malignant forms is problematic. Many studies should be done and moleculer techniques should be designed to overcome this dilemma.

6. References

Adrenal glands In: Basic histology 7th ed. Appleton and Lange, 1992:403-410

Adrenal gland and other paraganglia. In:Rosai and Ackerman's Surgical Pathology, 9th ed. Mosby, 2004:1115-1162

Arias-Stella J, Valcarcel J. (1973). The human carotid body at high altitudes. *Pathol Microbiol* , Vol.39, pp. 292-297

DeLellis RA, Suchow E, Wolfe HJ. Ultrastructure of nuclear inclusions in pheochromocytoma and paraganglioma. Hum Pathol 1980;11:205-207

DeLellis RA, Mangray S. The adrenal glands. In: Sternberg's Diagnostic Surgical Pathology, 4th ed. Philadelphia: LWW, 2004:621-667

DeLellis RA, Lloyd RV, Heitz PU, Eng C. Tumors of endocrine organs. Lyon: IARC Press,2004

Dobbie JW, Symington T. The human adrenal with special reference to vasculature. J Endocrinol 1966:34;479-489

Endocrine system In:Histology for Pathologists, 3rd ed. Philadelphia: LWW, 2007: 1167-1211

Fawcett DW, Long JA, Jones AL. The ultrastructure of endocrine glands. Recent Prog Horm Res 1969;25:315-318

Grynszpan-Winograd O. Ultrastructure of the chromaffin cell. In: Greep RO, Astwood EB, eds. Handbook of physiology. Washington, DC: American physiological society, 1975:295-308

Guresci S, Kara C, Ertugrul DT, Unsal A. Combined adrenal medullary hyperplasia and myelolipoma: a mimicker of phaeochromocytoma. Turkısh Jour Endoc Metab 2009;13:84-86

Hayes WS, Davidson AJ, Grimley PM, Hartman DS. Extraadrenal retroperitoneal paraganglioma:clinical pathologic and CT findings. Am J Roentgenol.1990:155;1247-1250

Ishay A, Dharon M, Luboshitzky R. Combined adrenal myelolipoma and medullary hyperplasia. Horm Res 2004;62:23-26

Lack EE, Travis WD, Oertel JE Adrenal cortical neoplasms . In: Lack EE ed. Pathology of adrenal glands Churchill Living Stone, New York, 1990: 115-171

Landes SK, Leigh C, Bonsib SM, Layne K. Occurence of melanin in phaeochromocytoma. Mod Pathol 1993;6:175-178

Li M, Wenig BM. Adrenal oncocytic pheochromocytoma. Am J Surg Pathol 2000;24:1552-1557

Linnoila RI, Keiser HR, Steinberg SM, Lack E Histopathology of benign versus malignant sympathoadrenal paragangliomas : clinicopathologic study of 120 cases including unusual histologic features. Hum Pathol 1990;21:1168-1180

McNicol AM. Update on tumors of the adrenal cortex, phaeochromocytoma and extra-adrenal paraganglioma Histopathology. 2011 Jan;58(2):155-68.

Page DL, DeLellis RA, Hough AJJ. Tumors of the adrenal, 2nd ed. Armed Forces Institute of Pathology: Washington DC, 1984

Pick L. Das Ganglioma embriyonale sympathicum. Klin Wochensrv 1912;49:16-22

ReMine WH, Chong Gc, Van Heerden Ja, Sheps Sg, Harrison EGJr. Current management of phaeochromocytoma Ann Surg 1974;179:740-748

Sclafani LM, Woodruff JM, Brennan MF. Extraadrenal retroperitoneal paragagliomas: natural history and responce to treatment Surgery 1990:108;1124-1129

Strong VE, Kennedy T, Al-Ahmedie H et al. Prognostic indicators of malignancy in adrenal pheochromocytomas: clinical,histopathologic, and cell cycle/apoptosis gene expression analysis. Surgery 2008:143;759-768

Thompson LD. Pheochromocytoma of the Adrenal gland Scaled Score (PASS) to seperate benign from malignant neoplasms: a clinicopathologic and immunophenotypic study of 100 cases. Am J Surg Pathol 2002: 26; 551-566

Tischler AS, DeLellis RA, Biales B, Nunnemacher G, Carabba VWolfe HJ. Nerve growth factor-induced neurite overgrowth from normal human chromaffin cells. Lab Invest 1980;43:399-409

Tumors of the adrenal gland. In: diagnostic histopathology of tumors, 3rd ed. Churchill Livingstone, 2007:1099-1122

Unger PD, Cohen JM, Thung SN, Gordon R, Pertsemlidis D, Dikman SH. Lipid degeneration in a pheochromocytoma histologically mimicking an adrenal cortical tumor. Ach Pathol Lab Med 1990;114:892-894

Unger P, Hoffman K, Pertsemlides D, Thung SN, Wolfe D, Kaneko M. S100 protein-positive sustentacular cells in malignant and locally aggressive adrenal pheochromocytomas. Ach Pathol Lab Med 1991;115:484-487

Wong DL. Epinehrine biosynthesis: hormonal and neural control during stress. Cell Mol Neurobiol 2006:26;891-900

Part 2

Pathophysiology 2. Study Experimental Models

3

Mouse Models of Human Familial Paraganglioma

Louis J. Maher III et al.[1]
Department of Biochemistry and Molecular Biology, Mayo Clinic, Rochester, MN, USA

1. Introduction

Tumor suppressor genes (TSGs) protect normal cells from tumorigenesis (Lasko et al., 1991; Sherr, 2004). Except in cases of haploinsufficiency, heterozygosity for a non-functional TSG allele protects a cell from tumor formation because the functional TSG allele produces a functional protein. Loss of heterozygosity (LOH) is a mechanism by which the remaining wild type tumor suppressor allele is lost, resulting in tumor formation (Lasko et al., 1991; Sherr, 2004). Loss of TSG expression may also occur by epigenetic silencing. The probability of a "second hit" follows a Poisson distribution with the number of tumors and time of incidence being variable in heterozygous carriers (Shao et al., 1999).

Many TSGs have been identified. Such genes play roles in many cellular functions including cell cycle checkpoint control, mitogenic signaling pathways, protein turnover, DNA damage, hypoxia and other stress responses (Sherr, 2004). Surprisingly, the *SdhB*, *SdhC*, and *SdhD* subunits of the metabolic enzyme succinate dehydrogenase (SDH), have also been identified as TSGs for neuroendocrine tumors such as paraganglioma (PGL) and pheocheomocytoma (PHEO).

PGLs are rare (1:300,000) tumors of neuroectodermal origin derived from paraganglia, a diffuse neuroendocrine system dispersed from the base of the skull to the pelvic floor (Baysal, 2002). PGLs are highly vascularized tumors that can originate in either the sympathetic or parasympathetic nervous systems (Baysal, 2002; Pacak et al., 2001).

Patients with PGL tumors that secrete catecholamines present symptoms of catecholamine excess including palpitations. The predominant clinical features of nonchromaffin PGLs are cranial nerve palsies and tinnitus; however, a small proportion of these nonchromaffin PGLs secrete catecholamines (Dluhy, 2002). A hereditary PGL predisposition is involved in at least 30% of cases (Maher & Eng, 2002; Bryant et al., 2003). Individuals with familial predisposition display at least 40% penetrance and a more severe presentation than those with the sporadic form of the disease. Extra-adrenal pheochromocytomas are estimated to be malignant in 40% of cases (Young et al., 2002). There is currently no effective cure for malignant PGL.

---

[1]Emily H. Smith[1], Emily M. Rueter[1], Nicole A. Becker[1], John Paul Bida[1], Molly Nelson-Holte[1], José Ignacio Piruat Palomo[2], Paula García-Flores[2], José López-Barneo[2] and Jan van Deursen[1]
1 Department of Biochemistry and Molecular Biology, Mayo Clinic, Rochester, MN, USA
2 Instituto de Biomedicina de Sevilla (IBiS), Hospital Universitario Virgen del Rocío/CSIC/Universidad de Sevilla, Sevilla, Spain

Five genes encoding subunits of the succinate dehydrogenase (SDH) complex (*SdhA, SdhB, SdhC,* and *SdhD*) (Astuti et al., 2001; Baysal et al., 2000; Niemann & Muller, 2000; Burnichon et al.) or the enzyme responsible for *SdhA* flavination (Kaelin, 2009; Hao et al., 2009) have been identified as tumor suppressor genes in familial PGL. *Sdh* gene defects may also be the cause of sporadic head and neck PGLs where deletions at the same or closely related loci (11q13 and 11q22-23) are observed (Bikhazi et al., 2000). The remaining half of familial PGLs result from inherited mutations associated with von Hippel-Lindau (VHL) syndrome, multiple endocrine neoplasia type 2 (MEN 2), or neurofibromatosis genes (Inabnet et al., 2000; Bryant et al., 2003).
The SDH complex catalyzes the oxidation of succinate (Su) to fumarate (Fu) in the tricarboxylic acid (TCA) cycle and delivers the resulting electrons through various carriers to the ubiquinone pool of the electron transport chain. These electrons are ultimately donated to oxygen to generate water in the process that forms a proton gradient across the inner mitochondrial membrane for ATP production. The porcine SDH complex (Fig. 1) has been studied by X-ray crystallography (Sun et al., 2005). The largest subunit, SdhA, is a flavoprotein of 70 kDa that contains the SDH active site and FAD moiety. A smaller subunit, SdhB is an iron-sulfur protein of 30 kDa carrying three dissimilar iron clusters, $[2Fe\text{-}2S]^{2+,1+}$, $[4Fe\text{-}4S]^{2+,1+}$, and $[3Fe\text{-}4S]^{1+,0+}$. *SdhA/B* are anchored to the membrane by *SdhC* and *SdhD* (15 kDa and 12.5 kDa, respectively), which coordinate a heme group and possess a ubiquinone binding site essential for electron transport into the respiratory chain.

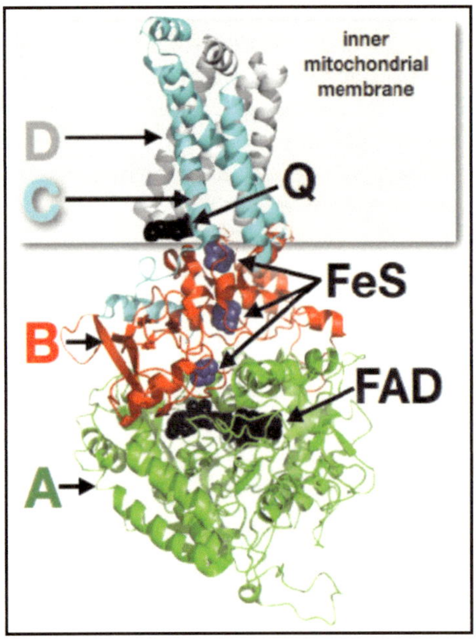

Fig. 1. X-ray crystal structure of SDH complex (Sun et al., 2005). Four subunits labeled and indicating the flavin of the catalytic A subunit (FAD), iron-sulfur clusters of the B subunit (FeS), and co-enzyme Q (Q) near the C and D subunits.

A broad spectrum of *Sdh* mutations has been reported in familial PGL. Mutations in *SdhB* and *SdhC* lead to non-imprinted autosomal dominant inheritance of familial PGL. Mutations in *SdhD* demonstrate imprinted paternal autosomal dominant inheritance (Baysal et al.,

2002). The range of mutations in SDH subunit genes identified in familial PGL suggests that loss of function of SDH subunits is the common cause of PGL.

Familial PGL is particularly fascinating because the causative genetic defects in SDH block the TCA cycle, enforcing upon the tumor an obligatory Warburg effect (Warburg, 1956). Thus, PGL tumor cells must apparently rely on glycolysis as an inefficient source of ATP. Familial PGL thus perfectly exemplifies the aerobic glycolysis commonly observed in cancer, and studies of PGL have the potential to reveal management strategies for all cancers that rely on glycolysis rather than the TCA cycle (Kaelin, 2009).

PGL causation may involve HIF1 activation and other epigenetic effects. Cells carefully regulate oxygen uptake, and respond to hypoxia by altering gene regulation. The master regulator of these responses is the heterodimeric basic helix-loop-helix transcription factor Hypoxia-Inducible Factor 1 (HIF1). HIF1 regulation involves oxygen-dependent prolylhydroxylation (PHD), ubiquitin ligation, and proteasomal degradation of the HIF1α subunit under normoxic conditions (Semenza, 2003). Prolylhydroxylation of HIF1α requires oxygen, iron, and 2-ketoglutarate (2KG), and the reaction produces succinate (Su) as a byproduct. If oxygen becomes limiting, prolylhydroxylation is inhibited, and HIF1α accumulates, translocates to the nucleus, and pairs with the constitutively expressed HIF1β subunit. Thus, HIF1 stability is directly regulated by oxygen. Hypoxic genes stimulated by HIF1 include transporters for increased glucose import (allowing anaerobic growth by glycolysis) and genes encoding angiogenesis factors. HIF1 activation is correlated with tumor aggressiveness and therapy resistance.

According to the succinate (Su) accumulation hypothesis (Lee et al., 2005; Maxwell, 2005; Selak et al., 2005; Smith et al., 2007; Favier & Gimenez-Roqueplo, 2010), the disruption of SdhB yields a catalytically inactive SdhA subunit and Su accumulates in the cell due to loss of SDH activity. Su diffuses to the cytoplasm where it acts as an inhibitor of the 2-ketoglutarate (2KG)-dependent prolyl hydroxylase (PHD) enzymes that use molecular oxygen as a substrate to hydroxylate HIF1α prolines for degradation when adequate oxygen is present. This class of enzyme reactions generates Su as a product, and is therefore susceptible to inhibition by elevated Su concentrations. Loss of SDH activity disables the TCA cycle and causes inappropriate HIF1 persistence due to Su inhibition of PHD enzymes. The resulting pseudohypoxic state is not tumorigenic in most cell types. However, it is hypothesized that chronic pseudohypoxic signaling is a mitogenic tumor initiator in neuroendocrine cells because these cells proliferate in a futile homeostatic attempt at a hormonal response to perceived hypoxia. Thus, inappropriate HIF1 persistence due to loss of SDH function in PGL drives tumorigenesis. HIF1 is therefore a novel target for therapy of PGL.

Our working hypotheses are shown in Fig. 2. We hypothesize that tumorigenic effects of succinate accumulation are not limited to inhibition of prolyl hydroxylation (McDonough et al., 2006), but also include inhibition of histone demethylation by Jumoni domain (JHDM) enzymes (Klose et al., 2006), and inhibition of 5-methylcytosine hydroxylation by TET1 (Tahiliani et al., 2009). Thus we are interested in model systems to probe how loss of SdhB acts as a tumorigenic trigger in neuroendocrine cells.

To date there have been limited opportunities to understand SDH dysfunction in such animal models. Although no human PGL cell lines exist, various studies have been undertaken using PGL tumor tissue samples to understand the underlying biochemistry and genetics (Benn et al., 2006). Unfortunately, such patient samples are not numerous and no systematic approach has been taken in understanding the pathological biochemistry of PGL.

Mutations in genes encoding *SdhB*, *SdhC*, or *SdhD* in *C. elegans*, *S. cerevisiae*, and mammalian cell lines have been utilized to examine the reactive oxygen species (ROS) hypothesis and the succinate accumulation hypothesis (Guo & Lemire, 2003; Ishii et al., 1998; Ishii et al., 2005; Lee et al., 2005; Oostveen et al., 1995; Selak et al., 2005). The only available mammalian PGL cell lines do not emulate the SDH familial form of PGL. For instance, rat PHEO cell line (PC12) (Tischler et al., 2004) and mouse PHEO cell lines (MPC) are available (Powers et al., 2000). However, PC12 cells are derived from a spontaneous PHEO tumor with functional Complex II and MPC cells are derived from neurofibromatosis [(*Nf1* +/- heterozygous] knockout mice (Tischler et al., 2004). During the course of this project a mouse model of *SdhD* deficiency was developed (Piruat et al., 2004). *SdhD* +/- mice were found to have decreased expression of *SdhD* and 50% SDH activity in various tissues relative to *SdhD* +/+ mouse tissues (Piruat et al., 2004). Although *SdhD* +/- mice were found to have carotid body glomus cell hyperplasia and organ hypertrophy, no PGL tumor formation was observed (Piruat et al., 2004; Bayley et al., 2009).

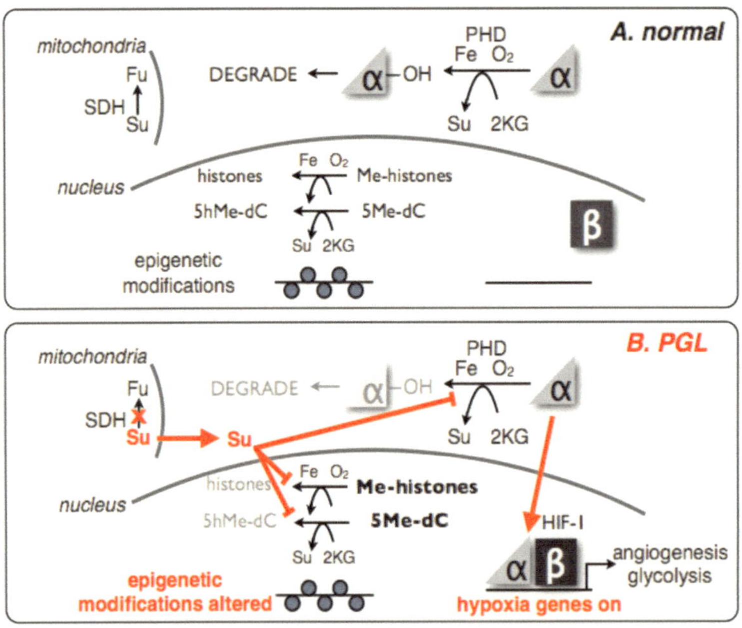

Fig. 2. A. Normal tumor suppressor functions of Fe/O_2/2KG-dependent dioxygenases in Hif-1α degradation and epigenetic regulation of histone methylation and 5-methylcytosine hydroxylation. B. Proposed effects of succinate inhibition in PGL. Simple genetic models of *Sdh* mutant PGL come in the form of model organisms that contain defects in SDH subunits.

We recently created and studied a yeast model lacking the *SdhB* subunit of Complex II (Smith et al., 2007). As expected for loss of a TCA enzyme, this yeast strain is dependent on glycolysis and is unable to survive on non-fermentable carbon sources. The yeast model has increased ROS and also shows accumulation of succinate. This succinate accumulation poisons at least two 2KG-dependent enzymes that produce succinate as a normal byproduct. Succinate inhibition of such enzymes in mammalian systems (e.g. the 2KG-dependent prolyl hydroxylase that modifies HIF-1α and JHDMs) has been proposed as a completely novel metabolic mechanism of tumorigenesis. Further progress in understanding PGL and PHEO could be facilitated by development of animal models to allow testing of the ROS and succinate accumulation hypotheses and hypotheses related to environment, diet, and pharmaceutical interventions.

Human *SdhB* mutations are not associated with a parent-of-origin effect (Baysal, 2001). It has also been observed that both *SdhB*- and *SdhD*-linked PGL tumors tend to lose *SdhB* expression and have enhanced *SdhA* abundance (Douwes Dekker et al., 2003). Thus, *SdhB* disruption creates an obvious goal for genetic models. Analysis of causative *SdhB* mutations in human PGL suggests that total loss of *SdhB* function is the common feature (Baysal, 2001; Baysal, 2002; Eng et al., 2003).

Here we describe the generation of two heterozygous mouse lines carrying a disruption in one copy of *SdhB*. By analogy with human familial predisposition to PGL genetics (Baysal, 2001; Baysal, 2002), mouse strains heterozygous for functional *SdhB* are hypothesized to display no phenotype, but to be predisposed to PGL development due to random loss of the second *SdhB* allele during development. Based on human PGL genetics, it was hypothesized that loss of the second *SdhB* gene would be oncogenic only in neuroendocrine cells.

2. Materials and methods

2.1 Creation of an *SdhB* targeting vector

A recombinant targeting vector for mouse *SdhB* was designed and assembled according to standard procedures. *SdhB*-specific sequences were inserted into the commercial vector NTKV1901 (Stratagene) that carries *Neo* and *TK* genes for selection of targeted integrants. Briefly, two arms homologous to segments of the murine *SdhB* gene were amplified by PCR (Epicentre, Failsafe kit) from mouse genomic DNA with sets of primers containing two unique restriction sites. The left homologous arm (Scrambler A) was PCR-amplified with an upstream primer that contains a *Hin*dIII site, (LJM-2309: $GCTAGCA_2GCT_2G_2AGATA$-$CAGCTCAGTCTGAGTG_3$) and a downstream primer that contains a *Xho*I site, (LJM-2310: $GCTAGC_2TCGAGCATC_2A_2CAC_2ATAG_2TC_2GCAC_2T$). The Scrambler A PCR product was directly cloned into the targeting vector NTKV1901. The right homologous arm (Scrambler B) was PCR-amplified with an upstream primer containing a *Cla*I site (LJM-2311: $GCTAGCATCGATG_2TG_2TGTC_2TGCTGTGCTGT_3GG$) and a downstream primer containing a *Sac*II site (LJM-2312: $GCTAGC_3GCG_4A_3G_2TG_4CAGACATAGTAC$). The Scrambler B PCR product was first cloned into a pGEM-T Easy vector (Promega), then isolated with a *Sac*II digest and ligated into the targeting vector. Diagnostic *Not*I, *Hin*dIII/*Xho*I and *Sac*II restriction digests were performed.

2.2 Extension the *SdhB* targeting vector

A forward primer specific for *SdhB* intron seven that contains the *Sal*I restriction site (LJM-2599: $ATATGTG_2TCAGTGCT_4C$) and a reverse primer specific for a region downstream of *Sdh*B exon eight that contains a *Not*I restriction site (LJM-2595: $GCTAGCGCG_2$-$C_2GC_2TA_2CTCACG_2A_2G_3CA_2G_2$) were used to amplify a Scrambler B extension product by PCR (Epicentre, Failsafe kit). The product was cloned into the original targeting vector using standard procedures.

2.3 ES cell culture and transfection with targeting vectors

ES cells derived from C57BL/6 blastocysts (E3.5) were transfected with *Not*I linearized targeting vectors, and stable integrants were selected in Geneticin G418 medium as described (Hofker & van Deursen, 2002).

2.4 Southern blotting

PCR was used to generate a 200-bp probe with homology to intron two of the *SdhB* gene. The probe was labeled by random priming in the presence of [α-^{32}P]-dATP according to manufacturer's instructions (Roche). 10-20 µg of genomic DNA from ES cell clones was digested with *Sac*I (New England Biolabs) and the DNA was electrophoresed overnight at 40 V. Southern blotting of DNA was performed using standard procedures as described (Hofker & van Deursen, 2002).

2.5 Genetic analysis of 129SV/E *SdhB:β-Geo* disrupted ES cells

For expression analysis by RT-PCR RNA was harvested from *SdhB* +/- ES cells with Trizol reagent by standard procedures, and reverse transcribed with a pool of nonamers according to manufacturer's instructions (Epicentre). cDNA was amplified with a common forward primer specific to *SdhB* exon one (LJM-2684: $CGACG_2TCG_3TCTC_2T_2GA_2$) and either a *β-Geo*-specific reverse primer (LJM-2687: $AT_2CAG_2CTGCGCA_2CTGT_2G_3$) or an exon two-specific reverse primer (LJM-2685: GAGCTGCAGCAGCAGCTGTC) by PCR (Epicentre, Failsafe kit). For mapping of the gene integration point by PCR genomic DNA from *SdhB* +/- ES cells was precipitated with lysis/precipitation buffer [50 mM Tris-HCl (pH 8.0), 100 mM EDTA (pH 8.0), 100 mM NaCl, 1% SDS, 10 mg/ml proteinase K] and extracted with phenol:chloroform (1:1). A forward primer specific for *SdhB* exon one (LJM-2784: $AGCTGAC_2AGACA_2GAGTCACAG_2TGAT_2GACAGA$) and a reverse primer specific for the *β-Geo* marker (LJM-2787: $AGTATCG_2C_2TCAG_2A_2GATCGCACTC_2AGC_2AGC$) were used to amplify the region of the gene trap vector integration by PCR (Epicentre, Failsafe kit). The PCR product was purified and sequenced across the *β-Geo* marker to verify the exact *SdhB:β-Geo* junction.

2.6 Generation and husbandry of mice

Following genetic characterization, *SdhB* +/- ES cells were injected into C57/BL6 blastocysts and used to generate chimeric animals as described (Hofker & van Deursen, 2002). Animals were caged in groups of five, segregated by genotype and gender. Standard animal husbandry methods were used under IACUC protocol A29505 in the Mayo Clinic non-barrier mouse facility.

2.7 DNA extraction

DNA extraction from tail clippings was performed after overnight digestion in lysis/precipitation buffer [50 mM Tris-HCl (pH 8.0), 100 mM EDTA (pH 8.0), 100 mM NaCl, 1% SDS, 10 mg/ml proteinase K] at 55°C. DNA was precipitated with isopropanol, washed once in 80% ethanol and resuspended in sterile water.

2.8 Genotyping

To distinguish *SdhB* +/+ and *SdhB* +/- animals, genomic DNA was analyzed by PCR (Epicentre, Failsafe kit) with a common forward primer LJM-2826 (5'-

$GTGTAGC_3TG_2CTGTC_2TG_2A_2CT_2GCTC$) and differential reverse primers, LJM-2828 (5'-$G_2CA_3C_3A_4G_3TCT_3GAGCAC_2AG$) and LJM-2830 (5'-$GTG_3AC_2TGCGTGACA_3GT GCATG_2AG$), specific for *β-Geo* and intron one, respectively. *Bub1* Genotyping used standard PCR methods employing the Failsafe kit (Epicentre). The *Bub1* WT locus was amplified with a forward primer in exon eight (LJM-3169: $CTG_2C_2TG_2A_2CT_2GCTATGTC$) and a reverse primer in intron eight (LJM-3171: $CG_2T_3CTCTGTATAGC_3TG_2C$). The *Bub1* knockout allele was amplified with a forward primer in the neomycin cassette (LJM-3178: $GCAGT_2CAT_2CAG_3CAC_2G_2AC$) and the reverse primer LJM-3171. The *Bub1* hypomorphic allele was amplified with a primer set in the hygromycin cassette (forward primer, LJM-3172: $CG_2A_2GTGCT_2GACAT_2G_2$; reverse primer, LJM-3173: $GTAT_2GAC_2GA$-$T_2C_2T_2GCG$).

2.9 Histology

Tissue samples for histology were dissected and fixed in neutral-buffered 10% formalin (Sigma) for 24 h. Tissues were dehydrated, embedded in paraffin, and 10-µm slices were prepared with a microtome and mounted. Standard hematoxylin and eosin staining was used for initial histopathology. Bifurcations containing carotid bodies were dissected and fixed in formalin (Sigma) at 4°C for 16 h. Tissues were dehydrated and paraffin embedded, and 10-µm slices were obtained by using an RM2125 microtome (Leica Microsystems). Immunohistochemistry was performed according to standard procedures. For detection of glomus cells, tissues were immunostained with a rabbit polyclonal antityrosine hydroxylase (TH) antibody (Pel-Freez). After immunodetection with peroxidase-conjugated secondary antibody, tissue samples were counterstained with hematoxylin.

2.10 Quantitative RNA analysis by RT-PCR

RNA from liver or kidney tissue was harvested with the RNeasy Plus Mini kit (Qiagen), quantitated with a RiboGreen assay (Invitrogen) and reverse transcribed by random nonamers (Epicentre). cDNA was amplified by PCR (BioRad IQ SuperMix) with a forward primer (LJM-3115: $ATGA_2CATCA_2CG_2AG_2CA_2TAC$) and a reverse primer (LJM-3116: $GAG_3TAGAT_4G_2AGACT_3GC$) located downstream of the βGEO insertion site in exon four. Probe 5'-6-FAM/$CACACGCAG_2ATCGACACG_2AC_2T$/3BHQ-1 specific for exon four was used to monitor target amplification of either cDNA or an 82-bp synthetic DNA amplicon used to produce a standard curve in a BioRad iCycler.

2.11 Enzyme assays

SDH activity was assayed in kidney and liver extracts from juvenile mice of each genotype euthanized by cervical dislocation. SDH activity was measured as PMS-mediated reduction of the 2,6-dichloroindophenol dye in the presence of antimycin A, rotenone and cyanide, monitored at 600 nm as described (Kramer et al., 2005).

2.12 Metabolite analysis

Levels of TCA cycle metabolites were determined by acidification of urine and extraction of free acids into ethyl acetate. 2-keto acids (e.g. 2-KG) were first protected by oximation with hydroxylamine hydrate. After evaporation, the dry residue was silyated with N,O-bis-(trimethylysilyl)trifluoroacetamide and trimethylchlorosilane to produce volatile derivatives, and analyzed by capillary gas chromatography/mass spectrometry on an HP ChemStation instrument equipped with an HP-5 25 m column (ID 0.2 mm) using pentadecanoic acid as an internal standard. Metabolite levels were normalized to creatine.

3. Results

3.1 Generation of *SdhB* +/- mice

Two approaches were initially taken to generate an *SdhB* +/- mouse strain (Fig. 3). The first strategy involved the creation of a DNA targeting vector that would specifically replace part of exon three through part of intron four by homologous recombination with a neomycin resistance marker on a single *SdhB* allele (Fig. 3A). The targeting vector carried two arms of homology to *SdhB* (Scrambler A and Scrambler B) and two selectable markers - NEO (neomycin phosphotransferase) and TK (thymidine kinase) genes. These genes allow for selection of integrants and counterselection against non-homologous insertions, respectively. This construct was intended to exchange the selectable NEO marker for a segment of *SdhB* extending from part of exon 3 through part of intron 4. This strategy would create an *SdhB* mRNA with only a short reading frame, followed by nonsense codons. The resulting truncated polypeptide is analogous to loss-of-function products seen in human *SdhB* mutations causing PGL (Benn et al., 2006).

The targeting vector was constructed and verified with diagnostic restriction digests that confirmed the successful insertion and orientation of both *SdhB* homology regions into the targeting vector. Its size (13.6 kb) was confirmed by linearization with *Not*I, Scrambler A insertion was confirmed by a *Hin*dIII/*Xho*I digest, and Scrambler B insertion was confirmed by a *Sac*II digest. Molecular junctions were sequenced to confirm expected features of the targeting vector.

Mouse ES cells were electroporated with the linearized *SdhB* targeting vector, and NEO+ TK- colonies were selected and screened for targeted inactivation of one copy of *SdhB*. DNA was harvested from over 400 potential clones and analyzed by Southern blot. None of the clones showed evidence of homologous recombination at *SdhB*. Similar results were obtained even when the Scrambler B *SdhB* homology segment was increased in length.

We therefore adopted a second strategy (Fig. 3B). We obtained an *SdhB* +/- embryonic stem (ES) cell line that had been created by high throughput random gene trap integration by the Sanger Center gene trap consortium (Nord et al., 2006). Sequencing of an RT-PCR product derived from the integrated *β-Geo* marker gene revealed integration of the gene trap cassette in intron 1 of the mouse *SdhB* gene. The strong cleavage and poly(A) signals of the gene trap fragment should truncate *SdhB* mRNA after the short exon 1, resulting in a completely non-functional *SdhB* mRNA, analogous to that produced by disease-associated truncating alleles in humans. We confirmed the presence of the gene trap by PCR from random-primed cDNA prepared from the ES cells. PCR of genomic DNA from the ES cell line allowed us to map the precise location of the gene trap, and sequencing of PCR products showed the exact position of the trap reporter gene downstream of the exon 1/intron 1 junction (Fig. 4A).

The *SdhB* +/- ES cells were injected into blastocyts that were then implanted in pseudopregnant females. Multiple chimeric offspring were obtained, four of which transmitted the mutant *SdhB* allele in their germ lines. These founders were mated with C57BL/6 strain females. A PCR screening procedure was developed (Fig. 4B) to allow genotyping of (129SV/E x C57BL/6)F1 offspring generated from *SdhB* +/+ x chimeric *SdhB* +/- matings. This approach proved successful for generating the desired *SdhB* +/- mouse strain used to develop a colony of 55 *SdhB* +/+ and 55 *SdhB* +/- mice.

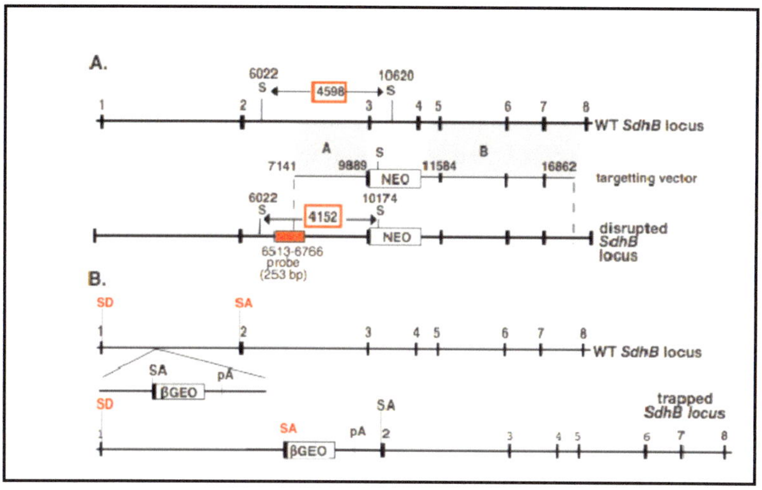

Fig. 3. *SdhB* knockout strategies. A. Targeted knockout approach. A targeting vector with homology regions encompassing intron two through part of exon three (shaded A) and encompassing part of intron four through intron seven (shaded B) flanking a neomycin cassette was used to target the WT *SdhB* locus and generate a disrupted *SdhB* locus. Numbers indicate position in *SdhB* locus from transcription start site. B. Gene trap vector approach. Gene trap vector contains a splice acceptor (SA) site upstream of the βGEO cassette (encodes β-galactosidase–neomycin phosphotransferase fusion protein) followed by a strong polyadenylation (pA) site inserted into intron one of *SdhB*. The SA site of the βGEO cassette will replace the SA site of exon two and will be spliced with the splice donor site of exon one.

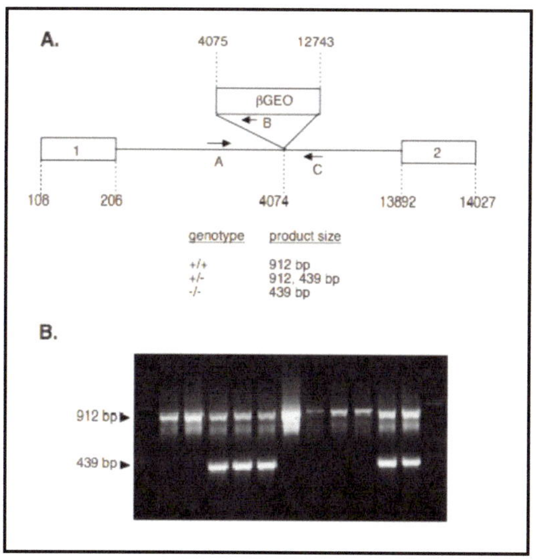

Fig. 4. *SdhB* genotyping PCR design. A. Schematic diagram showing the *SdhB* locus with or without a βGEO insertion in intron one. Primer set A/C amplifies the 912 bp WT locus and primer set A/B amplifies 439 bp from the disrupted locus. Numbers indicate position from the transcription start site in the wild type *SdhB* locus. B. PCR genotyping agarose gel showing *SdhB* +/+ vs. *SdhB* +/- amplification products from genomic DNA.

3.2 Characterization of *SdhB* +/- mice

We determined the viability of *SdhB* -/- mice. We hypothesized that the *SdhB* -/- condition would not support mammalian development due to lack of TCA cycle function. To test this hypothesis we crossed *SdhB* +/- heterozygotes and examined the genotypes of progeny. In the absence of *SdhB* -/- offspring, the prediction from Mendelian genetics is tbat 1/3 of progeny will be *SdhB* +/+ WT and 2/3 will be *SdhB* +/- heterozygotes. Breeding to test this hypothesis was performed until 107 offspring were genotyped. These offspring included 35 *SdhB* +/+ mice, 72 *SdhB* +/- mice with no *SdhB*(-/-) mice observed. This result implies that the *SdhB* -/- condition has an embryonic lethal phenotype. Indeed, it was previously reported that *SdhD* -/- mice die at 6.5 to 7.5 days post conception (Piruat et al., 2004). Evidence suggests that *SdhB* -/- mice also die around the time of organogenesis.

SdhB +/- mouse tissues were then characterized in terms of *SdhB* gene expression and SDH enzyme activity (Fig. 5).

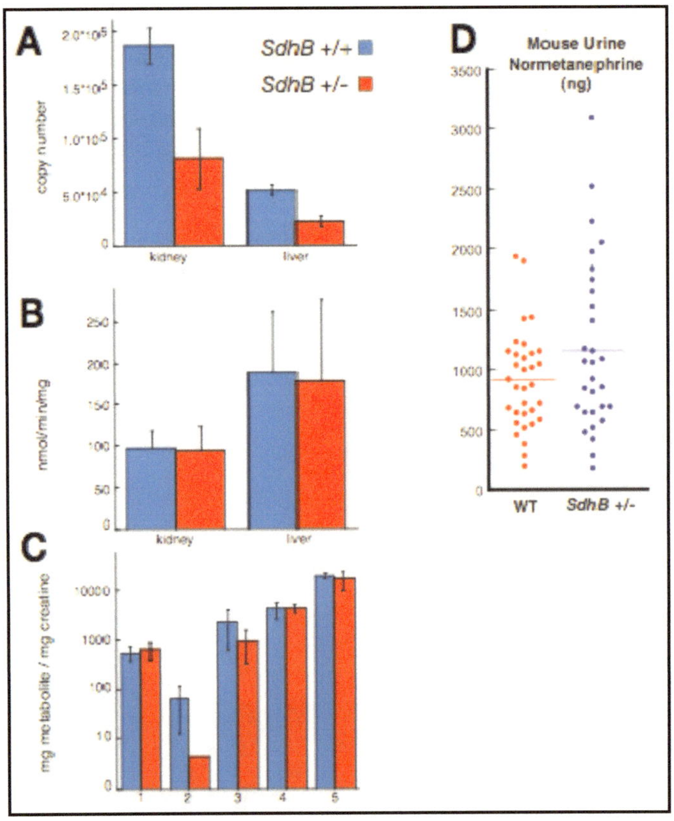

Fig. 5. Characterization of *SdhB* +/+ and *SdhB* +/- mice. A. *SdhB* expression levels (n=5). B. SDH activity (n=5). C. TCA metabolite levels in urine (n=3). 1, succinate; 2, fumarate; 3, malate; 4, citrate; 5, aconitate. Error basis indicates SEM. D. Results of 24-h urine normetanephrine screening in WT and *SdhB* +/- mice.

It was previously reported that *SdhD* +/- mice have a 50% decrease in *SdhD* expression and SDH activity (Piruat et al., 2004). We characterized *SdhB* expression and SDH activity in the liver and kidneys of *SdhB* +/- mice relative to *SdhB* +/+ mice. These organs have high metabolic activity and are easily homogenized for assays. We found that *SdhB* gene expression was decreased by 50% (based on quantitative RT-PCR analysis; Fig. 5A). In contrast, no difference in SDH enzyme activity was detected in these tissues (Fig. 5B), suggesting translational compensation or other homeostatic mechanisms. Furthermore, TCA cycle metabolites (He et al., 2004) in tissue (Fig. 5C) and metanephrines in urine (Fig. 5D) were not different between mice with *SdhB*+/+ and *SdhB*+/- genotypes.

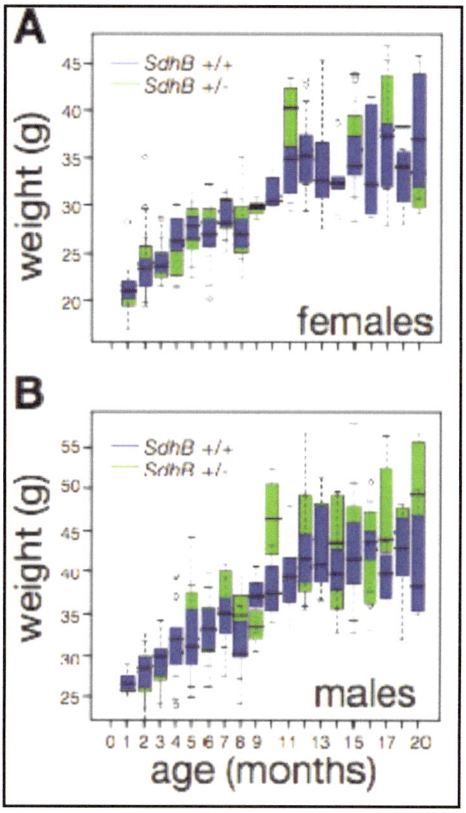

Fig. 6. Weight analysis for *SdhB* +/+ and *SdhB* +/- mice, by gender: A. Females. B. Males. The box represents the middle 50% of the weights (25-75%) and the horizontal bar represents the median weight for each group. The dashed lines encompass the remainder of the data, excluding outliers represented by circles.

Animals in the experimental colony were monitored by abdominal palpation and weight measurement. No abnormalities were detected in *SdhB* +/- animals. No significant differences were observed for weights of *SdhB* +/+ and *SdhB* +/- mice (Fig. 6). After one year, six *SdhB* +/+ and six *SdhB* +/- mice were euthanized and reviewed for gross and microscopic pathology of adrenal glands, heart, liver, lung, and kidneys. A detailed pathological analysis of carotid bodies investigated the possibility of neuroendocrine cell hypertrophy as has been suggested for *SdhD* +/- heterozygotes (Piruat et al., 2004). The results are shown in Fig. 7. Although there was a trend towards smaller carotid body size in *SdhB* +/- heterozygotes (Fig. 7A), the trend was not statistically significant (p values > 0.05 by t-test). This trend came mainly from male mice. Neuroendocrine cells of the carotid bodies of males were detected by tyrosine hydroxylase (TH) staining. Again, a trend toward a reduced number of type I (TH+) cells was observed in the *SdhB* +/- carotid bodies (Fig. 7B). Again, this difference was not statistically significant. There was no carotid body hypertrophy or any sign of hyperproliferation (Fig. 7C). No PGL or PHEO tumors were observed in any mice, even in compound *SdhB* +/- *SdhD* +/- heterozygotes.

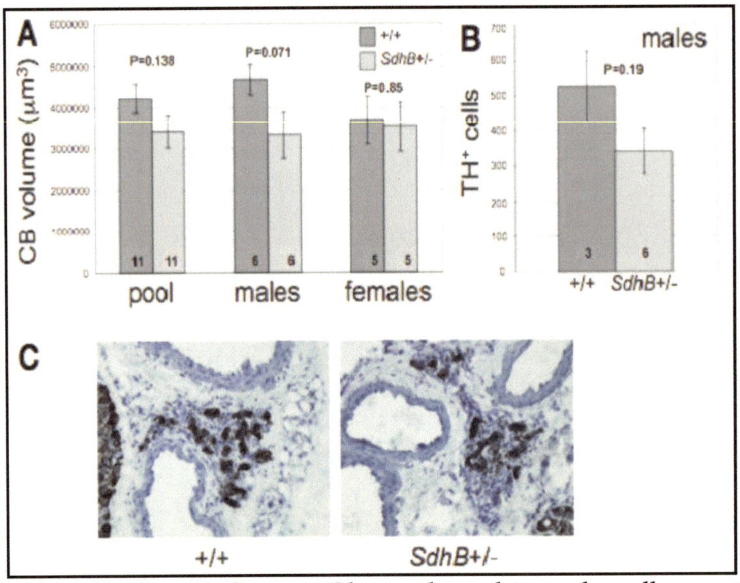

Fig. 7. Mouse carotid body pathology. A. Observed trend toward smaller carotid body size in *SdhB* +/- mice, not reaching statistic significance by t-test. The contribution to this trend comes mainly from males. B. Analysis of tyrosine hydroxylase positive (TH+) cells in carotid bodies from males. The trend toward a reduced number of TH+ cells in *SdhB* +/- male mice does not reach statistical significance. C. Examples of carotid body pathology. There is no evidence of carorid body hypertrophy or hyperproliferation in *SdhB* +/- mice.

3.3 Generation of *SdhB* +/- *Bub1* H/- mice

We hypothesized that the absence of PGL in *SdhB* +/- mice was due to the low rate of *SdhB* LOH. We therefore sought genetic methods to enhance this rate. Aneuploidy (abnormal chromosome content) is a hallmark of most solid tumors and cancer cell lines (Heim & Mitelman, 1995; Lengauer et al., 1997; Lengauer et al., 1997). Over 100 years ago Theodor Boveri postulated that chromosome instability (CIN) drives tumorigenesis. CIN is believed to be frequently responsible for TSG LOH (Bignold et al., 2006; Kops et al., 2005). More than 100 CIN genes have been identified in yeast (Kolodner et al., 2002; Nasmyth, 2002; Shonn et al., 2000). A novel mammalian gene of this type is *Bub1* (mouse chromosome 2), which plays a key role in the mitotic checkpoint.

Mitotic checkpoint proteins survey proper kinetichore attachment during mitosis. When the mitotic spindle is correctly attached to all kinetochores, Cdc20 activates the anaphase promoting complex (APC) to degrade securin, allowing release of separase to "unbind" sister chromatids and promote the transition from metaphase to anaphase (Kops et al., 2005). Mitotic checkpoint proteins produce a "stop anaphase" signal when kinetochores are not properly attached to the mitotic spindle during prometaphase. An APC inhibitory complex is involved (Kops et al., 2005; Shah & Cleveland, 2000; Wang et al., 2001). The BUB1 protein has three putative molecular functions in this mitotic checkpoint (Acampora et al., 1999) as illustrated in Fig. 8.

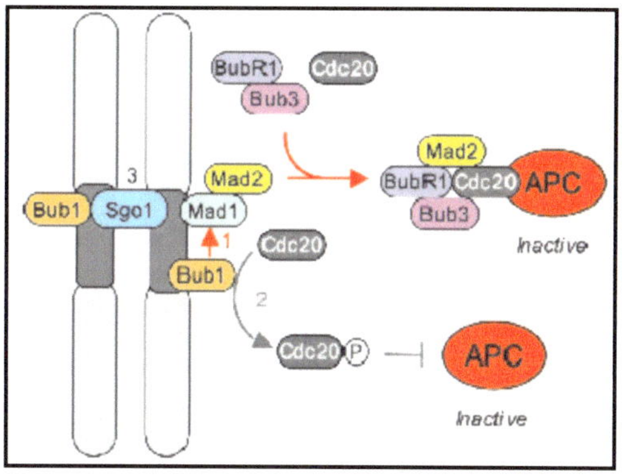

Fig. 8. Putative functions of *Bub1* in mitosis. 1. *Bub1* mediates Mad1/Mad2 binding to kinetochores, which allows for efficient formation of APC inhibitory complexes consisting of Mad2, BubR1, and Bub3. The APC inhibitory complex functions by sequestration of Cdc20. 2. *Bub1* phosphorylates Cdc20, thereby preventing APC activation. 3. *Bub1* is required for stability and centromeric localization of centromeric cohesin.

Loss of *Bub1* expression was predicted to result in aneuploidy and increased tumorigenesis. In support of this hypothesis, *Bub1* mutations were detected in 2/19 colorectal cancer cell lines with CIN (Cahill et al., 1998) and epigenetic silencing of *Bub1* is a frequent event in human colorectal carcinomas, with 30% exhibiting at least two-fold reduction in *Bub1* expression (Shichiri et al., 2002). In addition, *Bub1* mutations have been correlated with lung, pancreatic and rectal cancers (Gemma et al., 2000; Hempen et al., 2003; Imai et al., 1999).
The van Deursen laboratory has developed a series of mouse strains in which expression of *Bub1* protein is reduced in a graded fashion by different combinations of wild type, knockout, and hypomorphic alleles (Jeganathan et al., 2007). The *Bub1* hypomorphic allele [*Bub1*(H)] results from intron 9 insertion of the hygromycin B phosphotransferase gene (*Hyg*), resulting in a high level of premature transcription termination (van Deursen et al., 1994). Standard procedures and breeding yielded *Bub1* +/H, *Bub1* H/H, and *Bub1* H/- viable offspring. Western blotting showed graded reduction of *Bub1* levels across these strains in mouse embryonic fibroblasts.
Of the mice in the *Bub1* genotype series, the *Bub1* H/- strain shows the most dramatic phenotype. *Bub1* H/- mice display increased aneuploidy and tumorigenesis relative to the other *Bub1* genotypes. Analysis of 150 mitotic figures from *Bub1* H/- splenocytes showed 39% aneuploidy, compared to only 1% aneuploidy in *Bub1* +/+ animals (Jeganathan et al., 2007). *Bub1* H/- animals also suffer more tumors (52% tumor incidence in 530 days) than *Bub1* +/+ animals (33% tumor incidence in 772 days). Lymphoma and sarcoma incidence was higher and hepatocellular carcinoma incidence lower for *Bub1* H/- animals than for wild type animals.
Mutations in CIN genes can increase the rate of loss of entire chromosomes or chromosome segments during cell division, thereby accelerating LOH of tumor suppressor genes (Cahill et al., 1999; Cahill et al., 1998; Jallepalli & Lengauer, 2001). Indeed, it was shown in a cohort

of 30 *Bub1* H/- p53 +/- animals monitored for 100 days that 5 mice developed tumors. In contrast, 0/30 age-matched p53 +/- mice developed tumors during the same time period (Jeganathan et al., 2007). All tumors in *Bub1* H/- p53 +/- mice were thymic lymphomas, the most common tumor form in p53(-/-) mice (Donehower et al., 1992; Donehower et al., 1995; Jacks et al., 1994). Accelerated tumorigenesis resulted from p53 LOH as shown by PCR analysis of DNA from *Bub1* H/- p53 +/- lymphomas (Jeganathan et al., 2007; Jacks et al., 1994).

A two-part breeding program created a colony of 55 *SdhB* +/- *Bub1* H/- compound heterozygote mice (Fig. 9). In part 1, *SdhB* +/– females were crossed with *Bub1* H/- males to generate offspring of four genotypes (Fig. 9A). In part 2, offspring of these matings were crossed to generate the desired *SdhB* +/-*Bub1* H/- animals at the indicated expected frequencies (Fig. 9B). Multiplex PCR genotyping was developed to distinguish *Bub1* +, H and - alleles (Fig. 9C). The colony of *SdhB* +/- *Bub1* H/- compound heterozygote mice was monitored for PGL tumorigenesis. Age-dependent survival of this and related strains is shown in Fig. 10. As had been observed for *SdhB* +/- mice, no PGL tumors were observed in *SdhB* +/- *Bub1* H/- animals.

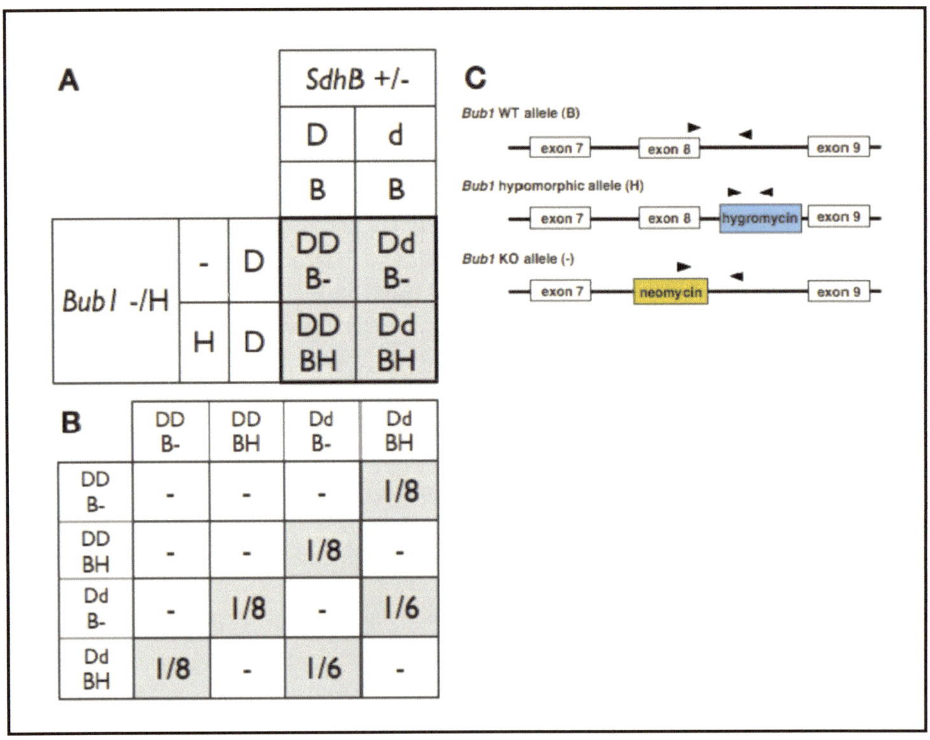

Fig. 9. *SdhB* +/- *Bub1* H/- breeding scheme. A. Initial cross providing offspring for brother-sister matings. B. Brother-sister mating scheme from (A), indicating expected frequencies of the desired *SdhB* +/- *Bub1* H/- genotype among offspring. Allele abbreviations: *SdhB* WT: D; *SdhB* gene trap disruption: d; *Bub1* WT: B; *Bub1* hypomorph, H; *Bub1* disruption: (-). C. *Bub1* Genotyping PCR design. Schematic diagram showing the *Bub1* locus with or without a hygromycin (hypomorphic allele) or neomycin (knockout allele) insertion. Primers used to amplify the alleles are designated by arrowheads.

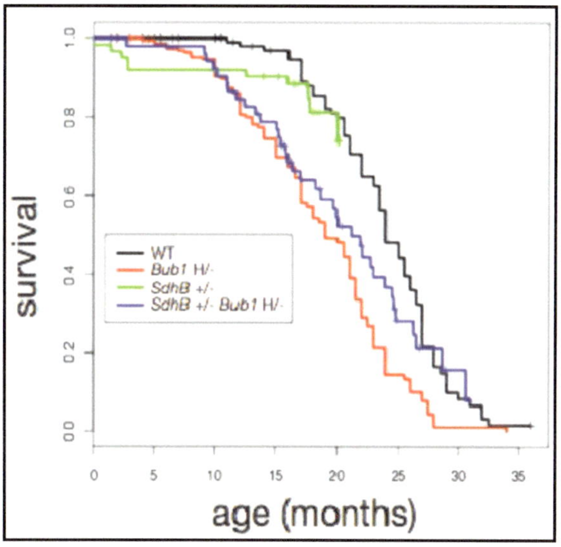

Fig. 10. Kaplan-Meier plot of mouse survival data.

4. Discussion

Spontaneous PGL is rare in mice (Jacks et al., 1994; Jacks et al., 1994). In a mouse model of human neurofibromatosis type 1, a dominant disease caused by inheritance of a mutant allele of NF1, a modest incidence of PHEO was observed (Jacks et al., 1994), but this genetic pathway to PGL appears unrelated to tumor suppression by *Sdh* genes.

We hypothesized that *SdhB* +/- mice would be predisposed to familial PGL. This hypothesis was based on the prevailing evidence that the *SdhB* +/- genotype predisposes humans to PGL, with high penetrance. We therefore developed a strain of *SdhB* +/- mice using mouse stem cells carrying a gene trap insertion in intron 1 of *SdhB*. Using these animals we showed that, as anticipated, the *SdhB* -/- genotype is not viable. Although we found that there is a significant reduction of SdhB expression in tissues of *SdhB* +/- mice relative to *SdhB* +/+ mice, there was no difference in SDH activity between the two groups in either liver or kidney. These results suggest that there is no phenotypic difference between *SdhB* +/- and *SdhB* +/+ mice, consistent with the absence of phenotype for humans heterozygous for *Sdh* germline mutations. However, unlike humans where there is high penetrance of PGL in *SdhB* +/- individuals, no PGL tumors were detected in *SdhB* +/- mice.

LOH of a TSG can be the rate-limiting step in tumor development (Lasko et al., 1991; Luo et al., 2000). The mechanism for LOH is not completely understood but involves chromosome loss, deletion and/or homologous interchromosomal mitotic recombination events (Henson et al., 1991; Shao et al., 2000; Stark & Jasin, 2003). Mitotic recombination refers to the reciprocal exchange of genetic material between nonsister chromatids in mitotic cells. Mitotic recombination occurs at a high frequency in humans and mice (Gupta et al., 1997; Holt et al., 1999; Shao et al., 1999). It has been suggested that mitotic recombination is the predominant pathway to LOH (Gupta et al., 1997; Luo et al., 2000; Shao et al., 1999; Shao et al., 2000).

Because mitotic recombination requires high nucleotide sequence homology, chromosomal divergence suppresses mitotic recombination and may modify cancer development by lowering the rate of LOH (Shao et al., 2001). The use of inbred strains in this study (C57BL/6 x 129SVE)F1 should promote mitotic recombination. It has also been found that the spontaneous frequency of mitotic recombination increases with age (Grist et al., 1992). The penetrance of *SdhB* mutations in familial PGL is estimated to be 50% at age 30 and approaches 100% after 60 years of age (Neumann et al., 2004).

To address the possible limitation of LOH in converting somatic neuroendocrine cells from *SdhB* +/- to *SdhB* -/-, we developed a mouse colony of *SdhB* +/- mice bred onto the *Bub1* H/- genetic background previously shown to enhance aneuploidy. PGL tumorigenesis was not observed in this strain.

There are at least three possible explanations for these results. First, it is possible that the rate of somatic LOH at *SdhB* in neuroendocrine cells remains insufficient to drive PGL tumorigenesis within the lifespan of mice. Second, it is possible that PGL tumorigenesis takes place in *SdhB* +/- mice, but the subsequent rate of tumor growth is too slow to permit tumor detection within the mouse lifespan. Finally, it is possible that *SdhB* is not a tumor suppressor in murine PGL.

If either of the first two explanations are correct, it might be possible to enhance the rate of PGL tumorigenesis by developing a conditional knockout mouse strain where both copies of the *Sdh* gene for one SDH subunit are replaced by a knock-in construct that can be recombinationally inactived upon expression of a recombinase. Unlike standard conditional knock-out designs, it would be important to delete the *Sdh* subunit gene only at very low frequency, since most affected tissues would presumably be damaged by loss of the TCA cycle. Rather, an inefficient recombination that eliminated SDH in perhaps 1% of cells might be appropriate. This might be achieved either by low levels of neuroendocrine-specific expression of recombinase (e.g. from the tyrosine hydroxylase promoter), or by low levels of global recombinase expression. Unfortunately, mouse strains are not yet available for tissue-specific CRE expression in neuroendocrine cells.

Either low-efficiency conditional knockout strategy offers the prospect of dramatically increasing the early generation of neuroendocrine cells lacking SDH activity. Such a model would be hypothesized to increase the frequency of tumorigenesis, and allow a longer period for tumor growth.

5. Acknowledgments

We acknowledge the technical assistance of Ming Li, Wei Zhou, Darren Baker, Molly van Norman, Piero Rinaldo, Ron Marler, and Leslie Dixon in the generation and analysis of knockout animals. This work was supported by the Mayo Foundation, the Mayo Graduate School, and by a grant from the Fraternal Order of Eagles.

6. References

Acampora, D., V. Avantaggiato, F. Tuorto, P. Barone, M. Perera, D. Choo, D. Wu, G. Corte, and A. Simeone. (1999). Differential Transcriptional Control as the Major Molecular Event in Generating Otx1-/- and Otx2-/- Divergent Phenotypes. *Development*. Vol. 126, no. 7, pp. 1417-26.

Astuti, D., F. Latif, A. Dallol, P. L. Dahia, F. Douglas, E. George, F. Skoldberg, E. S. Husebye, C. Eng, and E. R. Maher. (2001). Gene Mutations in the Succinate Dehydrogenase Subunit Sdhb Cause Susceptibility to Familial Pheochromocytoma and to Familial Paraganglioma. *American Journal of Human Genetics*. Vol. 69, no. 1, pp. 49-54.

Bayley, J.-P., I. van Minderhout, P.C.W. Hogendoorn, C.J. Cornelisse, A. van der Wal, F.A. Prins, L. Teppema, A. Dahan, P. Devilee, P.E.M. Taschner. (2009). *Sdhd* and *Sdhd/H19* Knockout Mice do not Develop Paraganglioma or Pheochromocytoma. PLoS ONE. Vol. 4, no. 11, e7987.

Baysal, B. E. (2001). Genetics of Familial Paragangliomas: Past, Present, and Future. *Otolaryngology Clinics of North America*. Vol. 34, no. 5, pp. 863-79, vi.

Baysal, B. E.. (2002). Hereditary Paraganglioma Targets Diverse Paraganglia. *Journal of Medical Genetics*. Vol. 39, no. 9, pp. 617-22.

Baysal, B. E., R. E. Ferrell, J. E. Willett-Brozick, E. C. Lawrence, D. Myssiorek, A. Bosch, A. van der Mey, P. E. Taschner, W. S. Rubinstein, E. N. Myers, C. W. Richard, 3rd, C. J. Cornelisse, P. Devilee, and B. Devlin. (2000). Mutations in *SdhD*, a Mitochondrial Complex II Gene, in Hereditary Paraganglioma. *Science*. Vol. 287, no. 5454, pp. 848-51.

Baysal, B. E., J. E. Willett-Brozick, E. C. Lawrence, C. M. Drovdlic, S. A. Savul, D. R. McLeod, H. A. Yee, D. E. Brackmann, W. H. Slattery, 3rd, E. N. Myers, R. E. Ferrell, and W. S. Rubinstein. (2002). Prevalence of Sdhb, Sdhc, and Sdhd Germline Mutations in Clinic Patients with Head and Neck Paragangliomas. *Journal of Medical Genetics*. Vol. 39, no. 3, pp. 178-83.

Benn, D. E., A. P. Gimenez-Roqueplo, J. R. Reilly, J. Bertherat, J. Burgess, K. Byth, M. Croxson, P. L. Dahia, M. Elston, O. Gimm, D. Henley, P. Herman, V. Murday, P. Niccoli-Sire, J. L. Pasieka, V. Rohmer, K. Tucker, X. Jeunemaitre, D. J. Marsh, P. F. Plouin, and B. G. Robinson. (2006). Clinical Presentation and Penetrance of Pheochromocytoma/Paraganglioma Syndromes. *Journal of Clinical Endocrinology and Metabolism*. Vol. 91, no. 3, pp. 827-36.

Bignold, L. P., B. L. Coghlan, and H. P. Jersmann. (2006). Hansemann, Boveri, Chromosomes and the Gametogenesis-Related Theories of Tumours. *Cell Biology International*. Vol. 30, no. 7, pp. 640-4.

Bikhazi, P. H., L. Messina, A. N. Mhatre, J. A. Goldstein, and A. K. Lalwani. (2000). Molecular Pathogenesis in Sporadic Head and Neck Paraganglioma. *Laryngoscope*. Vol. 110, no. 8, pp. 1346-8.

Bryant, J., J. Farmer, L. J. Kessler, R. R. Townsend, and K. L. Nathanson. (2003). Pheochromocytoma: The Expanding Genetic Differential Diagnosis. *Journal of the National Cancer Institute*. Vol. 95, no. 16, pp. 1196-204.

Burnichon, N., J. J. Briere, R. Libe, L. Vescovo, J. Riviere, F. Tissier, E. Jouanno, X. Jeunemaitre, P. Benit, A. Tzagoloff, P. Rustin, J. Bertherat, J. Favier, and A. P. Gimenez-Roqueplo. *SdhA* Is a Tumor Suppressor Gene Causing Paraganglioma. *Human Molecular Genetics*. Vol. 19, no. 15, pp. 3011-20.

Cahill, D. P., K. W. Kinzler, B. Vogelstein, and C. Lengauer. (1999). Genetic Instability and Darwinian Selection in Tumours. *Trends in Cell Biology*. Vol. 9, no. 12, pp. M57-60.

Cahill, D. P., C. Lengauer, J. Yu, G. J. Riggins, J. K. Willson, S. D. Markowitz, K. W. Kinzler, and B. Vogelstein. (1998). Mutations of Mitotic Checkpoint Genes in Human Cancers. *Nature*. Vol. 392, no. 6673, pp. 300-3.

Dluhy, R. G. (2002). Pheochromocytoma--Death of an Axiom. *New England Journal of Medicine*. Vol. 346, no. 19, pp. 1486-8.

Donehower, L. A., M. Harvey, H. Vogel, M. J. McArthur, C. A. Montgomery, Jr., S. H. Park, T. Thompson, R. J. Ford, and A. Bradley. (1995). Effects of Genetic Background on

Tumorigenesis in P53-Deficient Mice. *Molecular Carcinogenesis*. Vol. 14, no. 1, pp. 16-22.

Donehower, L.A., M. Harvey, B.L. Slagle, M.J. McArthur, C.A. Montgomery, Jr., J.S. Butel, and A. Bradley. (1992). Mice Deficient for p53 Are Developmentally Normal but Susceptible to Spontaneous Tumours. *Nature*. Vol. 356, 215-21.

Douwes Dekker, P. B., P. C. Hogendoorn, N. Kuipers-Dijkshoorn, F. A. Prins, S. G. van Duinen, P. E. Taschner, A. G. van der Mey, and C. J. Cornelisse. (2003). *SdhD* Mutations in Head and Neck Paragangliomas Result in Destabilization of Complex II in the Mitochondrial Respiratory Chain with Loss of Enzymatic Activity and Abnormal Mitochondrial Morphology. *Journal of Pathololog*y. Vol. 201, no. 3, pp. 480-6.

Eng, C., M. Kiuru, M. J. Fernandez, and L. A. Aaltonen. (2003). A Role for Mitochondrial Enzymes in Inherited Neoplasia and Beyond. *Nature Reviews Cancer*. Vol. 3, no. 3, pp. 193-202.

Favier, J., and A. P. Gimenez-Roqueplo. (2010). Pheochromocytomas: The (Pseudo)-Hypoxia Hypothesis. Best practice & research *Clinical Endocrinology and Metabolism*. Vol. 24, no. 6, pp. 957-68.

Gemma, A., M. Seike, Y. Seike, K. Uematsu, S. Hibino, F. Kurimoto, A. Yoshimura, M. Shibuya, C. C. Harris, and S. Kudoh. (2000). Somatic Mutation of the Hbub1 Mitotic Checkpoint Gene in Primary Lung Cancer. *Genes Chromosomes Cancer*. Vol. 29, no. 3, pp. 213-8.

Grist, S. A., M. McCarron, A. Kutlaca, D. R. Turner, and A. A. Morley. (1992). In Vivo Human Somatic Mutation: Frequency and Spectrum with Age. *Mutation Research*. Vol. 266, no. 2, pp. 189-96.

Guo, J., and B. D. Lemire. (2003). The Ubiquinone-Binding Site of the Saccharomyces Cerevisiae Succinate-Ubiquinone Oxidoreductase Is a Source of Superoxide. *Journal of Biological Chemistry*. Vol. 278, no. 48, pp. 47629-35.

Gupta, P. K., A. Sahota, S. A. Boyadjiev, S. Bye, C. Shao, J. P. O'Neill, T. C. Hunter, R. J. Albertini, P. J. Stambrook, and J. A. Tischfield. (1997). High Frequency in Vivo Loss of Heterozygosity Is Primarily a Consequence of Mitotic Recombination. *Cancer Research*. Vol. 57, no. 6, pp. 1188-93.

Hao, H. X., O. Khalimonchuk, M. Schraders, N. Dephoure, J. P. Bayley, H. Kunst, P. Devilee, C. W. Cremers, J. D. Schiffman, B. G. Bentz, S. P. Gygi, D. R. Winge, H. Kremer, and J. Rutter. (2009). Sdh5, a Gene Required for Flavination of Succinate Dehydrogenase, Is Mutated in Paraganglioma. *Science*. Vol. 325, no. 5944, pp. 1139-42.

He, W., F. J. Miao, D. C. Lin, R. T. Schwandner, Z. Wang, J. Gao, J. L. Chen, H. Tian, and L. Ling. (2004). Citric Acid Cycle Intermediates as Ligands for Orphan G- Protein-Coupled Receptors. *Nature*. Vol. 429, no. 6988, pp. 188-93.

Heim, S., and F. Mitelman. Cancer Cytogenetics. New York: Wiley-Liss Inc., 1995.

Hempen, P. M., H. Kurpad, E. S. Calhoun, S. Abraham, and S. E. Kern. (2003). A Double Missense Variation of the Bub1 Gene and a Defective Mitotic Spindle Checkpoint in the Pancreatic Cancer Cell Line Hs766t. *Human Mutation*. Vol. 21, no. 4, pp. 445.

Henson, V., L. Palmer, S. Banks, J. H. Nadeau, and G. A. Carlson. (1991). Loss of Heterozygosity and Mitotic Linkage Maps in the Mouse. *Proceedings of the National Academy of Sciences, USA*. Vol. 88, no. 15, pp. 6486-90.

Hofker, M.H., and J. vanDeursen, eds. Transgenic Mouse Methods and Protocols, Methods in Molecular Biology. Totowa, NJ: Humana Press, 2002.

Holt, D., M. Dreimanis, M. Pfeiffer, F. Firgaira, A. Morley, and D. Turner. (1999). Interindividual Variation in Mitotic Recombination. *American Journal of Human Genetics*. Vol. 65, no. 5, pp. 1423-7.

Imai, Y., Y. Shiratori, N. Kato, T. Inoue, and M. Omata. (1999). Mutational Inactivation of Mitotic Checkpoint Genes, Hsmad2 and Hbub1, Is Rare in Sporadic Digestive Tract Cancers. *Japanses Journal of Cancer Research*. Vol. 90, no. 8, pp. 837-40.

Inabnet, W. B., P. Caragliano, and D. Pertsemlidis. (2000). Pheochromocytoma: Inherited Associations, Bilaterality, and Cortex Preservation. *Surgery*. Vol. 128, no. 6, pp. 1007-11;discussion 11-2.

Ishii, N., M. Fujii, P. S. Hartman, M. Tsuda, K. Yasuda, N. Senoo-Matsuda, S. Yanase, D. Ayusawa, and K. Suzuki. (1998). A Mutation in Succinate Dehydrogenase Cytochrome B Causes Oxidative Stress and Ageing in Nematodes. *Nature*. Vol. 394, no. 6694, pp. 694-7.

Ishii, T., K. Yasuda, A. Akatsuka, O. Hino, P. S. Hartman, and N. Ishii. (2005). A Mutation in the Sdhc Gene of Complex Ii Increases Oxidative Stress, Resulting in Apoptosis and Tumorigenesis. *Cancer Research*. Vol. 65, no. 1, pp. 203-9.

Jacks, T., L. Remington, B. O. Williams, E. M. Schmitt, S. Halachmi, R. T. Bronson, and R. A. Weinberg. (1994). Tumor Spectrum Analysis in P53-Mutant Mice. *Current Biology*. Vol. 4, no. 1, pp. 1-7.

Jacks, T., T. S. Shih, E. M. Schmitt, R. T. Bronson, A. Bernards, and R. A. Weinberg. (1994). Tumour Predisposition in Mice Heterozygous for a Targeted Mutation in Nf1. *Nature Genetics*. Vol. 7, no. 3, pp. 353-61.

Jallepalli, P. V., and C. Lengauer. (2001). Chromosome Segregation and Cancer: Cutting through the Mystery. *Nature Reviews Cancer*. Vol. 1, no. 2, pp. 109-17.

Jeganathan, K., L. Malureanu, D. J. Baker, S. C. Abraham, and J. M. van Deursen. (2007). Bub1 Mediates Cell Death in Response to Chromosome Missegregation and Acts to Suppress Spontaneous Tumorigenesis. *Journal of Cell Biology*. Vol. 179, no. 2, pp. 255-67.

Kaelin, W. G. (2009). Sdh5 Mutations and Familial Paraganglioma: Somewhere Warburg Is Smiling. *Cancer Cell*. Vol. 16, no. 3, pp. 180-2.

Klose, R. J., E. M. Kallin, and Y. Zhang. (2006). Jmjc-Domain-Containing Proteins and Histone Demethylation. *Nature Reviews Genetics*. Vol. 7, no. 9, pp. 715-27.

Kolodner, R. D., C. D. Putnam, and K. Myung. (2002). Maintenance of Genome Stability in *Saccharomyces Cerevisiae*. *Science*. Vol. 297, no. 5581, pp. 552-7.

Kops, G. J., B. A. Weaver, and D. W. Cleveland. (2005). On the Road to Cancer: Aneuploidy and the Mitotic Checkpoint. *Nature Reviews Cancer*. Vol. 5, no. 10, pp. 773-85.

Kramer, K. A., D. Oglesbee, S. J. Hartman, J. Huey, B. Anderson, M. J. Magera, D. Matern, P. Rinaldo, B. H. Robinson, J. M. Cameron, and S. H. Hahn. (2005). Automated Spectrophotometric Analysis of Mitochondrial Respiratory Chain Complex Enzyme Activities in Cultured Skin Fibroblasts. *Clinical Chemistry*. Vol. 51, no. 11, pp. 2110- 6.

Lasko, D., W. Cavenee, and M. Nordenskjold. (1991). Loss of Constitutional Heterozygosity in Human Cancer. *Annual Reviews of Genetics*. Vol. 25, 281-314.

Lee, S., E. Nakamura, H. Yang, W. Wei, M. S. Linggi, M. P. Sajan, R. V. Farese, R. S. Freeman, B. D. Carter, W. G. Kaelin, and S. Schlisio. (2005). Neuronal Apoptosis Linked to Egln3 Prolyl Hydroxylase and Familial Pheochromocytoma Genes: Developmental Culling and Cancer. *Cancer Cell*. Vol. 8, no. 2, pp. 155-67.

Lengauer, C., K. W. Kinzler, and B. Vogelstein. (1997). DNA Methylation and Genetic Instability in Colorectal Cancer Cells. *Proceedings of the National Academy of Sciences USA*. Vol. 94, no. 6, pp. 2545-50.

Lengauer, C. (1997). Genetic Instability in Colorectal Cancers. *Nature*. Vol. 386, no. 6625, pp. 623-7.

Luo, G., I. M. Santoro, L. D. McDaniel, I. Nishijima, M. Mills, H. Youssoufian, H. Vogel, R. A. Schultz, and A. Bradley. (2000). Cancer Predisposition Caused by Elevated Mitotic Recombination in Bloom Mice. *Nature Genetics*. Vol. 26, no. 4, pp. 424-9.

Maher, E. R., and C. Eng. (2002). The Pressure Rises: Update on the Genetics of Phaeochromocytoma. *Human Molecular Genetics*. Vol. 11, no. 20, pp. 2347-54.

Maxwell, P. H. (2005). A Common Pathway for Genetic Events Leading to Pheochromocytoma. *Cancer Cell*. Vol. 8, no. 2, pp. 91-3.

McDonough, M. A., V. Li, E. Flashman, R. Chowdhury, C. Mohr, B. M. Li√©nard, J. Zondlo, N. J. Oldham, I. J. Clifton, J. Lewis, L. A. McNeill, R. J. Kurzeja, K. S. Hewitson, E. Yang, S. Jordan, R. S. Syed, and C. J. Schofield. (2006). Cellular Oxygen Sensing: Crystal Structure of Hypoxia-Inducible Factor Prolyl Hydroxylase (Phd2). *Proceedings of the National Academy of Sciences USA*. Vol. 103, no. 26, pp. 9814-9.

Nasmyth, K. (2002). Segregating Sister Genomes: The Molecular Biology of Chromosome Separation. *Science*. Vol. 297, no. 5581, pp. 559-65.

Neumann, H. P., C. Pawlu, M. Peczkowska, B. Bausch, S. R. McWhinney, M. Muresan, M. Buchta, G. Franke, J. Klisch, T. A. Bley, S. Hoegerle, C. C. Boedeker, G. Opocher, J. Schipper, A. Januszewicz, and C. Eng. (2004). Distinct Clinical Features of Paraganglioma Syndromes Associated with *SdhB* and *SdhD* Gene Mutations. *Journal of the American Medical Association*. Vol. 292, no. 8, pp. 943-51.

Niemann, S., and U. Muller. (2000). Mutations in *SdhC* Cause Autosomal Dominant Paraganglioma, Type 3. *Nature Genetics*. Vol. 26, no. 3, pp. 268-70.

Nord, A. S., P. J. Chang, B. R. Conklin, A. V. Cox, C. A. Harper, G. G. Hicks, C. C. Huang, S. J. Johns, M. Kawamoto, S. Liu, E. C. Meng, J. H. Morris, J. Rossant, P. Ruiz, W. C. Skarnes, P. Soriano, W. L. Stanford, D. Stryke, H. von Melchner, W. Wurst, K. Yamamura, S. G. Young, P. C. Babbitt, and T. E. Ferrin. (2006). The International Gene Trap Consortium Website: A Portal to All Publicly Available Gene Trap Cell Lines in Mouse. *Nucleic Acids Research*. Vol. 34, no. Database issue, pp. D642-8.

Oostveen, F. G., H. C. Au, P. J. Meijer, and I. E. Scheffler. (1995). A Chinese Hamster Mutant Cell Line with a Defect in the Integral Membrane Protein Cii-3 of Complex II of the Mitochondrial Electron Transport Chain. *Journal of Biological Chemistry*. Vol. 270, no. 44, pp. 26104-8.

Pacak, K., W. M. Linehan, G. Eisenhofer, M. M. Walther, and D. S. Goldstein. (2001). Recent Advances in Genetics, Diagnosis, Localization, and Treatment of Pheochromocytoma. *Annals of Internal Medicine*. Vol. 134, no. 4, pp. 315-29.

Piruat, J. I., C. O. Pintado, P. Ortega-Saenz, M. Roche, and J. Lopez-Barneo. (2004). The Mitochondrial Sdhd Gene Is Required for Early Embryogenesis, and Its Partial Deficiency Results in Persistent Carotid Body Glomus Cell Activation with Full

Responsiveness to Hypoxia. *Molecular and Cellular Biology*. Vol. 24, no. 24, pp. 10933-40.

Powers, J. F., M. J. Evinger, P. Tsokas, S. Bedri, J. Alroy, M. Shahsavari, and A. S. Tischler. (2000). Pheochromocytoma Cell Lines from Heterozygous Neurofibromatosis Knockout Mice. *Cell and Tissue Research*. Vol. 302, no. 3, pp. 309-20.

Selak, M. A., S. M. Armour, E. D. MacKenzie, H. Boulahbel, D. G. Watson, K. D. Mansfield, Y. Pan, M. C. Simon, C. B. Thompson, and E. Gottlieb. (2005). Succinate Links Tca Cycle Dysfunction to Oncogenesis by Inhibiting Hif-Alpha Prolyl Hydroxylase. *Cancer Cell*. Vol. 7, no. 1, pp. 77-85.

Semenza, G. L. (2003). Targeting Hif-1 for Cancer Therapy. *Nature Reviews Cancer*. Vol. 3, no. 10, pp. 721-32.

Shah, J. V., and D. W. Cleveland. (2000). Waiting for Anaphase: Mad2 and the Spindle Assembly Checkpoint. *Cell*. Vol. 103, no. 7, pp. 997-1000.

Shao, C., L. Deng, O. Henegariu, L. Liang, N. Raikwar, A. Sahota, P. J. Stambrook, and J. A. Tischfield. (1999). Mitotic Recombination Produces the Majority of Recessive Fibroblast Variants in Heterozygous Mice. *Proceedings of the National Academy of Sciences USA*. Vol. 96, no. 16, pp. 9230-5.

Shao, C., L. Deng, O. Henegariu, L. Liang, P. J. Stambrook, and J. A. Tischfield. (2000). Chromosome Instability Contributes to Loss of Heterozygosity in Mice Lacking p53. *Proceedings of the National Academy of Sciences USA*. Vol. 97, no. 13, pp. 7405-10.

Shao, C., P. J. Stambrook, and J. A. Tischfield. (2001). Mitotic Recombination Is Suppressed by Chromosomal Divergence in Hybrids of Distantly Related Mouse Strains. *Nature Genetics*. Vol. 28, no. 2, pp. 169-72.

Sherr, C. J. (2004). Principles of Tumor Suppression. *Cell*. Vol. 116, no. 2, pp. 235-46.

Shichiri, M., K. Yoshinaga, H. Hisatomi, K. Sugihara, and Y. Hirata. (2002). Genetic and Epigenetic Inactivation of Mitotic Checkpoint Genes *Hbub1* and *Hbubr1* and Their Relationship to Survival. *Cancer Research*. Vol. 62, no. 1, pp. 13-7.

Shonn, M. A., R. McCarroll, and A. W. Murray. (2000). Requirement of the Spindle Checkpoint for Proper Chromosome Segregation in Budding Yeast Meiosis. *Science*. Vol. 289, no. 5477, pp. 300-3.

Smith, E. H., R. Janknecht, and L. J. Maher, 3rd. (2007). Succinate Inhibition of {Alpha}-Ketoglutarate-Dependent Enzymes in a Yeast Model of Paraganglioma. *Human Molecular Genetics*. Vol. 16, no. 24, pp. 3136-48.

Stark, J. M., and M. Jasin. (2003). Extensive Loss of Heterozygosity Is Suppressed During Homologous Repair of Chromosomal Breaks. *Molecular and Cellular Biology*. Vol. 23, no. 2, pp. 733-43.

Sun, F., X. Huo, Y. Zhai, A. Wang, J. Xu, D. Su, M. Bartlam, and Z. Rao. (2005). Crystal Structure of Mitochondrial Respiratory Membrane Protein Complex II. *Cell*. Vol. 121, no. 7, pp. 1043-57.

Tahiliani, M., K. P. Koh, Y. Shen, W. A. Pastor, H. Bandukwala, Y. Brudno, S. Agarwal, L. M. Iyer, D. R. Liu, L. Aravind, and A. Rao. (2009). Conversion of 5-Methylcytosine to 5-Hydroxymethylcytosine in Mammalian DNA by Mll Partner Tet1. *Science*. Vol. 324, no. 5929, pp. 930-5.

Tischler, A. S., J. F. Powers, and J. Alroy. (2004). Animal Models of Pheochromocytoma. *Histology and Histopathology*. Vol. 19, no. 3, pp. 883-95.

van Deursen, J., W. Ruitenbeek, A. Heerschap, P. Jap, H. ter Laak, and B. Wieringa. (1994). Creatine Kinase (Ck) in Skeletal Muscle Energy Metabolism: A Study of Mouse Mutants with Graded Reduction in Muscle Ck Expression. *Proceedings of the National Academy of Sciences USA*. Vol. 91, no. 19, pp. 9091-5.

Wang, X., J. R. Babu, J. M. Harden, S. A. Jablonski, M. H. Gazi, W. L. Lingle, P. C. de Groen, T. J. Yen, and J. M. van Deursen. (2001). The Mitotic Checkpoint Protein Hbub3 and the mRNA Export Factor Hrae1 Interact with Gle2p-Binding Sequence (Glebs)-Containing Proteins. *Journal of Biological Chemistry*. Vol. 276, no. 28, pp. 26559-67.

Warburg, O. (1956). On the Origin of Cancer Cells. *Science*. Vol. 123, no. 3191, pp. 309-14.

Young, A. L., B. E. Baysal, A. Deb, and W. F. Young, Jr. (2002). Familial Malignant Catecholamine-Secreting Paraganglioma with Prolonged Survival Associated with Mutation in the Succinate Dehydrogenase B Gene. *Journal of Clinical Endocrinology and Metabolism*. Vol. 87, no. 9, pp. 4101-5.

4

Cell Differentiation Induction Using Extracellular Stimulation Controlled by a Micro Device

Yuta Nakashima[1], Katsuya Sato[2], Takashi Yasuda[3]
and Kazuyuki Minami[1]
[1]*Yamaguchi University*
[2]*The University of Tokushima*
[3]*Kyushu Institute of Technology*
Japan

1. Introduction

The stem cell differentiation is greatly dependent on the living environment *i.e.*, the cell differentiation determined by timing, amplitude, amount and etc. of stimulation from outside of cells (Lanza & Rosenthal, 2004). If living environment of cell can be controlled artificially by using micro device, we will be able to guide the cell having specific function from stem cells. The micromachining technology allows integration of various mechanical, electrical, and chemical elements, and has produced micro devices that can manipulate chemical solution, small mechanical parts, cells and etc. (Meyer et al., 2000; Takeuchi & Shimoyama, 1999; Nakashima et al., 2010; Nakashima & Yasuda, 2009; Chen et al., 2007; Taff & Voldman, 2005; Choi & Park, 2005; Doh & Cho, 2005). Our purpose is to fabricate micro devices which can control cell differentiation and axon elongation by extracellular stimulation. The cell differentiation induction on the micro devices will be applied to a technique for restoring impaired or lost biological function and controlling differentiation of a stem cell to a specific cell. This paper presents two micro devices intended to control the induction of cell differentiation dynamically by chemical stimulation and mechanical stimulation. First, we present a chemical stimulation device consisting of a microvalve, a nano-holes array, and a chamber, which are placed very close to one another. The amount of chemical solution released from the nano-hole array can be controlled very precisely by opening and closing the microvalve. Also, we show the behavior of cells stimulated using the fabricated chemical stimulation device, *i.e.*, differentiation guidance of cells using release control of nerve growth factor (NGF) which is a protein that enhances axonal outgrowth from a cell body. Next, we present a mechanical stimulation device consisting of a chamber for cell culture and a microlinkage mechanism for applying uniaxial stretching to the microchamber. Then we show the fluorescence observation of behavior of a cell that receives stimulation by fabricated mechanical stimulation device.

2. Chemical stimulation device

2.1 Design of the chemical stimulation device

The microdevice we designed for chemical stimulation consists of a nano-hole array for NGF release, a hydrophobic passive microvalve for controlling NGF release, a microchannel for carrying NGF and a chamber for cell culture as shown in Fig. 1(a, b) (Nakashima & Yasuda, 2005; Nakashima & Yasuda, 2009). The device is microfabricated from a SOI (Silicon on Insulator) wafer as detailed below. A chamber for cultivating a cell was fabricated on one side of the wafer, and a microchannel was fabricated on the other side. The nano-hole array was fabricated in a SiO_2 membrane of 0.5 μm in thickness. The inside diameter of the nano-holes must be less than 0.5 μm because the typical diameter of an axon terminal is 0.5 - 4 μm. The etching technique using FIB (Focused Ion Beam, Seiko Instruments Inc., JFIB-2300) satisfies the need for the fabrication of such small holes. Nerve cells are cultured on a SiO_2 diaphragm including the nano-hole array.

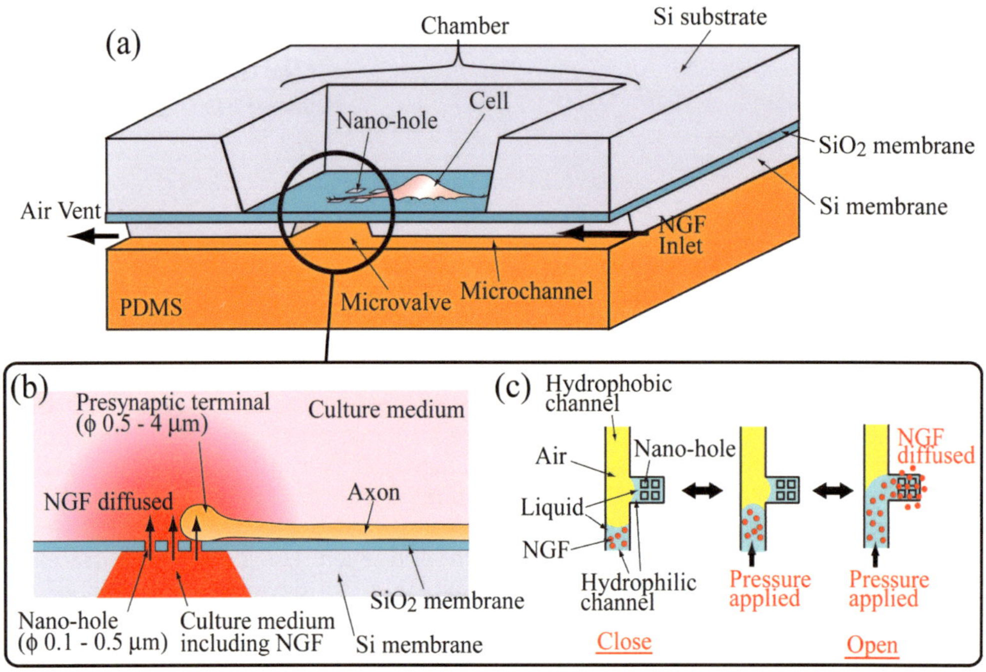

Fig. 1. Schematic of a fabricated chemical stimulation micro device.

Figure 1(c) shows the schematic of liquid switching principle of a microvalve using different liquid surface tensions on hydrophilic and hydrophobic channels. Liquids injected into the hydrophilic channels stop at the boundary between the hydrophilic and hydrophobic channels. The air that was initially in the hydrophobic channel separates the two liquids. When pressure is applied from the inlet, the inlet liquid will break into the hydrophobic channel and merge with the outlet liquid. If the inlet liquid includes NGF, it will diffuse into the outlet liquid. This is a hydrophobic passive microvalve which has very simple structure without any mechanically movable parts and which can be driven by low pressure (Yun et al, 2002; Lee et al, 2002).

Figure 2 shows the SEM photograph which was taken from the channel side of the device. The microchannel measures 60 μm in width and 8 μm in depth. 100 nano-holes with a square side of about 500 nm in length were opened in the SiO_2 membrane inside the channel. The microvalve was constructed at the T-shaped crossing of the microchannel.

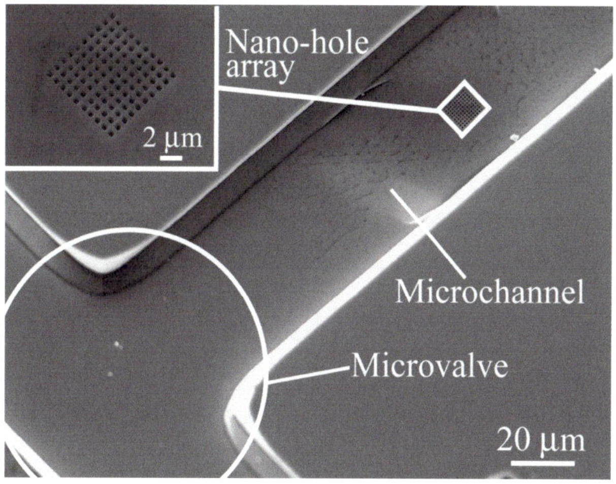

Fig. 2. SEM photographs of the fabricated device. The microchannels including a hydrophobic passive microvalve and nano-hole array.

2.2 Device fabrication

Figure 3 shows the fabrication process of the chemical stimulation device. SiO_2 films were created by thermal oxidation on both sides of a SOI wafer that consists of 350 μm thick handle Si layer, 500 nm thick SiO_2 layer, and 8 μm thick Si layer (Fig. 3(a)). The SOI wafer was spin-coated with photoresist ZPN-1150 (ZEON Corp.) on the front side, and the SiO_2 film was patterned by photolithography and wet etching. In order to fabricate the culture chamber, the thick Si layer was etched anisotropically (Fig. 3(b)). Next, the microchannel was fabricated by anisotropically etching the backside of Si layer (Fig. 3(c)). Then, the microvalve was fabricated by lift-off method of Au deposition and by creating hydrophobic SAM (self assembled monolayer), 1-octadecanethiol on the Au surface (Fig. 3(d)). The nano-holes were fabricated in a SiO_2 membrane by FIB (Fig. 3(e)). Finally, the culture chamber was coated by collagen, and the microchannels were covered with the PDMS sheet.

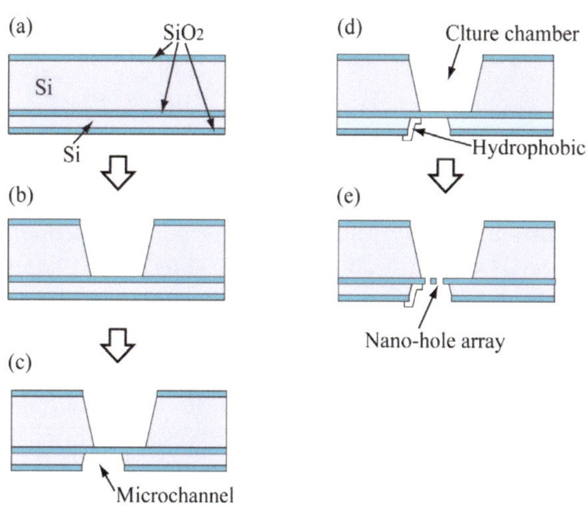

Fig. 3. Fabrication process of the chemical stimulation device.

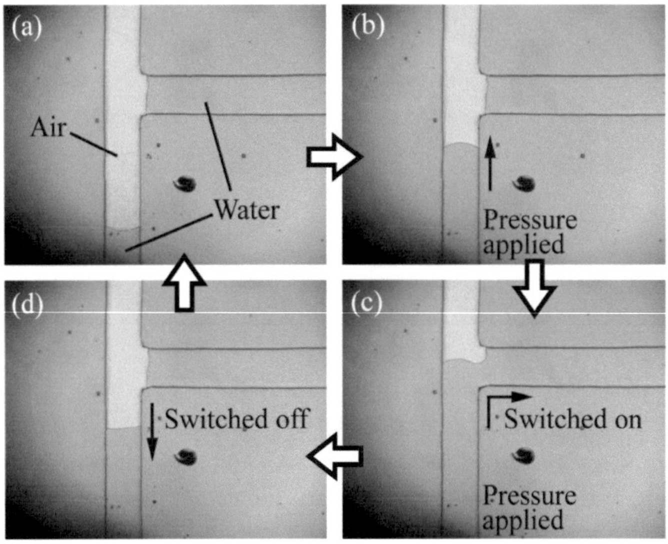

Fig. 4. Photograph of liquid switching test using the fabricated microvalve. (a) The initial state. (b) Inlet pressure was applied. (c) The valve opened. (d) The valve closed after eliminating inlet pressure.

2.3 Switching test of the microvalve and chemical release tests

Figure 4 shows the photograph of the test result using deionized water as the test liquid. When water was injected into the channel, it was infiltrated into the hydrophilic channel by the capillary force and stopped at the edge of the hydrophobic channel. Inlet water was initially separated from outlet water (Fig. 4(a)). When inlet pressure was applied, inlet water began to flow through the hydrophobic channel (Fig. 4(b)) and eventually merged with outlet water (Fig. 4(c)). When inlet pressure was eliminated, water stopped flowing and separated into two fluids. At the inlet, water flowed backwards (Fig. 4(d)) and returned to the original state (Fig. 4(a)). This enabled us to open and close the microvalve with inlet pressure. Also, we confirmed that when culture medium is used as a working fluid having higher viscosity than water, the fabricated microvalve could open and close.

2.4 Chemical release tests

Chemical release tests were conducted using the fabricated microfluidic device. We observed diffusion of the fluorescent dye (Rhodamine B, Molecular Probes, Inc., R-648) released through the nano-hole array under the inverted microscope (Nikon Co., TE2000). Figure 5 shows experimental setup for chemical release testing. When pressure was applied from the liquid inlet, a hydrophobic microvalve will open and the fluorescent dye oozed from the nano-hole array and spread out into the deionized water that filled the chamber of the device.

Figure 6 shows that the fluorescent dye was oozing from the nano-hole array and spreading out into the deionized water by diffusion. The fluorescence intensity was measured at several positions (see Figure 6(b)) at 60 sec after the diffusion began. The dye concentration decreased by 56 % at the position of 50 μm away from the nano-hole array as shown in Figure 7.

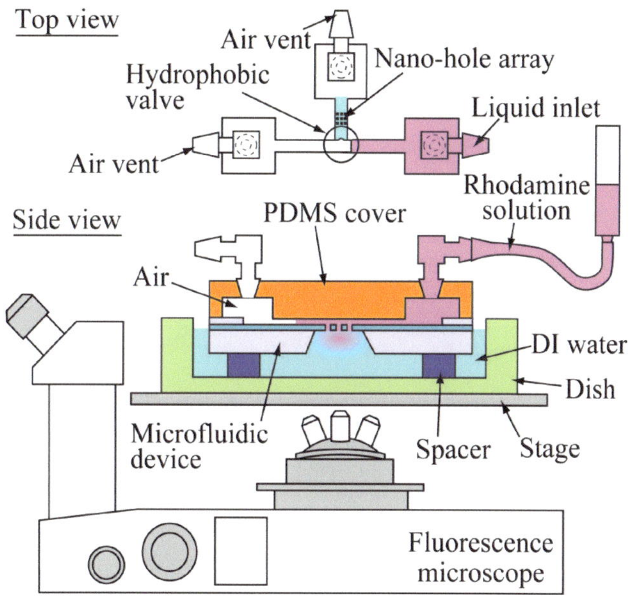

Fig. 5. Experimental setup. The fabricated microfluidic device was covered with PDMS film. Diffusion of the fluorescent dye through the nano-hole array was observed under the inverted microscope.

The variation in the fluorescence intensity synchronized with opening and closing of the microvalve as shown in Fig.8. The fluorescence intensity rose immediately after the valve opened, and decreased immediately when the valve was closed. Additionally, the fluorescence intensity changed according to the switching interval, the smaller the fluorescence intensity change. This result means that the fabricated device can control release of chemical solution by opening and closing of the valve.

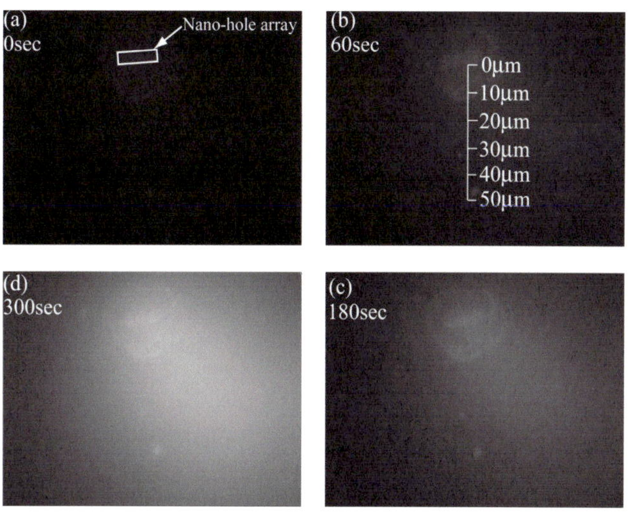

Fig. 6. Diffusion of fluorescent dye through a nano-hole array. Light gray indicates high concentration of fluorescent dye.

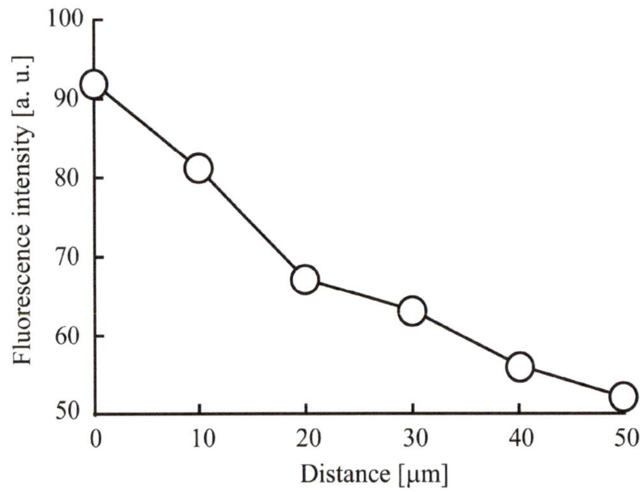

Fig. 7. Relationship between the fluorescence intensity and distance from the nano-hole at 60 sec after the diffusion began.

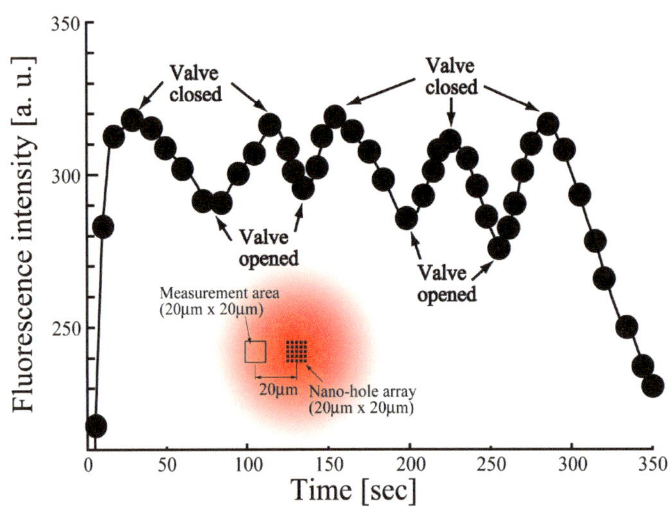

Fig. 8. Variation in the fluorescence intensity after the microvalve is opened and closed repeatedly.

2.5 Cell differentiation induction test by chemical stimulation

PC 12 (adrenal pheochromocytoma) cells were used in the experiments and prepared as follows. The cells were maintained in culture medium (RPMI1640, SIGMA-ALDRICH Corp.) supplemented with 10 % fetal bovine serum and 100 ng/ml nerve growth factor (NGF). The cells were cultured in 5 % CO_2 at 37 °C for 3 days to start their differentiation and make them sensitive to NGF stimulation. Then, these cells were collected by pipetting, and cultivated without NGF on the cell culture chamber of the fabricated device in 5 % CO_2 at 37 °C for 30 min. Finally, the cells were stimulated chemically by releasing NGF through the nano-hole array on the device.

We confirmed whether cell differentiation can be controlled on the device or not. Figure 9 shows experimental procedure for cell differentiation induction. Growth of cells stimulated by NGF is observed under a microscope from the chamber side. The inlet culture medium containing NGF and the culture medium in the cell culture chamber are initially separated by a closed hydrophobic microvalve. When pressure is applied from the inlet, the inlet liquid and the chamber liquid are connected by opening the microvalve. After that, NGF diffused into the chamber liquid and is released into the chamber through the nano-hole array. Thus, the cells in the chamber are stimulated by NGF.

We conducted the experiment that was NGF stimulation controlled by periodic switching of the microvalve using the fabricated microdevice. We observed the growth of cultured cells while the microvalve was switched at 1Hz under the inverted microscope. As shown in Fig.10, the lower left cell that adhered to the device surface elongated the axon toward nano-holes as time passed. On the other hand, because the right side cell did not adhere to the device surface at first, it could not begin to differentiate. However, after it succeeded in adhering to the device surface 2 hours after the original stimulus was applied, the right side cell also demonstrated our intended movement manner, *i.e.* it elongated the axon toward the nano-holes as time passed. From this result, we conclude that we can guide the cell differentiation and the axon elongation by the fabricated microdevice.

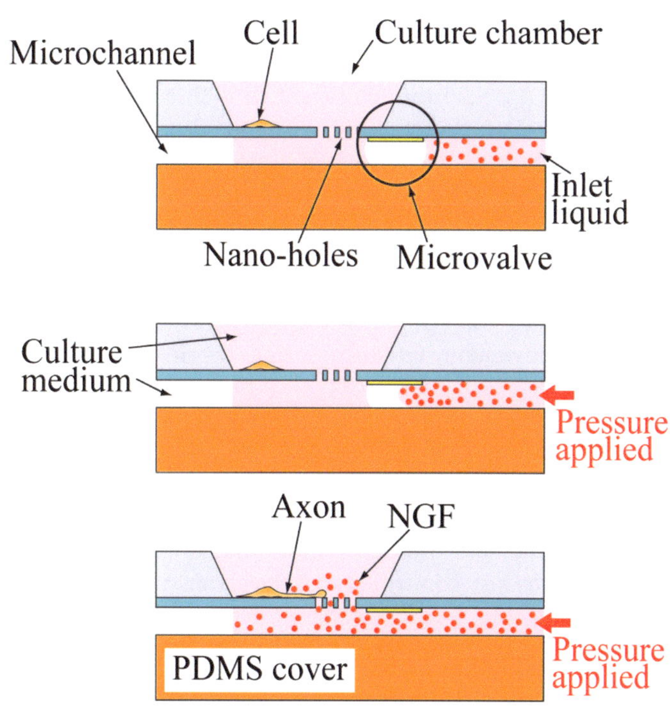

Fig. 9. Experimental procedure for cell differentiation induction using fabricated microdevice.

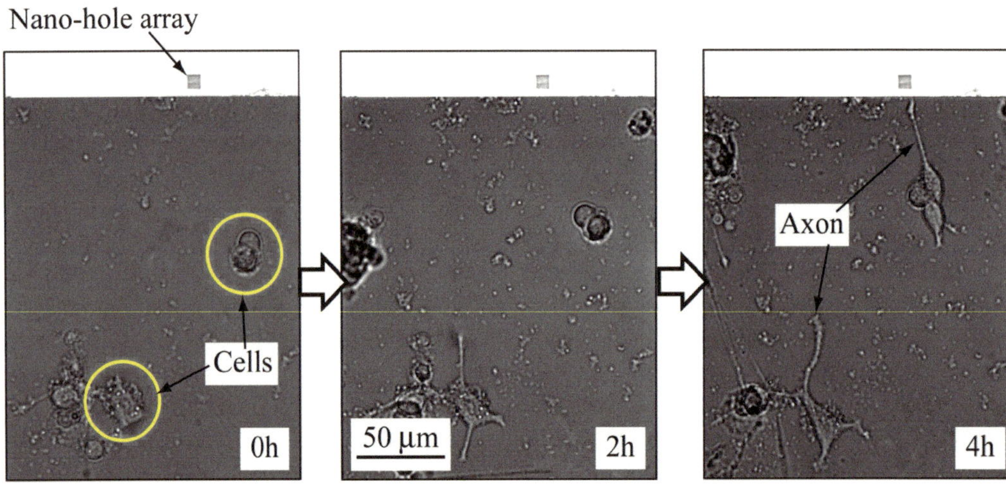

Fig. 10. Cell differentiation guidance on the fabricated microfluidic device. The axons elongated toward the nano-holes according to NGF stimulation from the nano-holes.

3. Mechanical stimulation device

3.1 Design of the mechanical stimulation device

The mechanical stimulation device developed in the present study is fabricated on a glass coverslip and 6 devices are fabricated on one coverslip. This coverslip with the microdevice is bonded to the bottom of a $\phi = 35$ mm culture dish with a 14 mm hole and used in the experiment. With this device, an inverted microscope and an oil-immersion objective lens can be used for the observation. The schematic of a mechanical stimulation device is shown in Fig. 11. The size of each device is 2 mm square. This device consists of one microchamber made of PDMS, one pair of stretching arms by which the microchamber is uniaxially stretched, the journal bearings that support the stretching arms, and the slider that drives the stretching arms (Sato et al., 2010). The slider is pushed by a microneedle connected to the micromanipulator that drives the pair of stretching arms. Finally, sliding movement is converted into rotation movement via the journal bearing, and the microchamber is stretched from each side.

Figure 12 shows the SEM photograph of the fabricated device. A micro three-dimensional structure was fabricated by multiple exposures to SU-8. The dimension error in the link mechanism was measured as approximately 5 μm. The clearance in the journal bearing and slider was designed to be 10 μm to allow the dimension error arise in the fabrication process, therefore, the journal bearing, the most important element in the link mechanism, was successfully fabricated. It was also confirmed that the slider was successfully fabricated and that all of the link mechanisms were movable structures. The chamber has a thin film stretching part (stretching substrate) in the center of the chamber. The size of the stretching substrate is 400 x 100 μm and the thickness is 10 μm. The stretching substrate is supported by the surrounding support frame with the size of 50 μm width and 50 μm thickness. The microchamber also has a binding part with stretching arms at both the ends of the support frame. In the fabrication process, six microchambers are molded on one glass coverslip at once. The excess part is cut and removed to obtain the chamber shape.

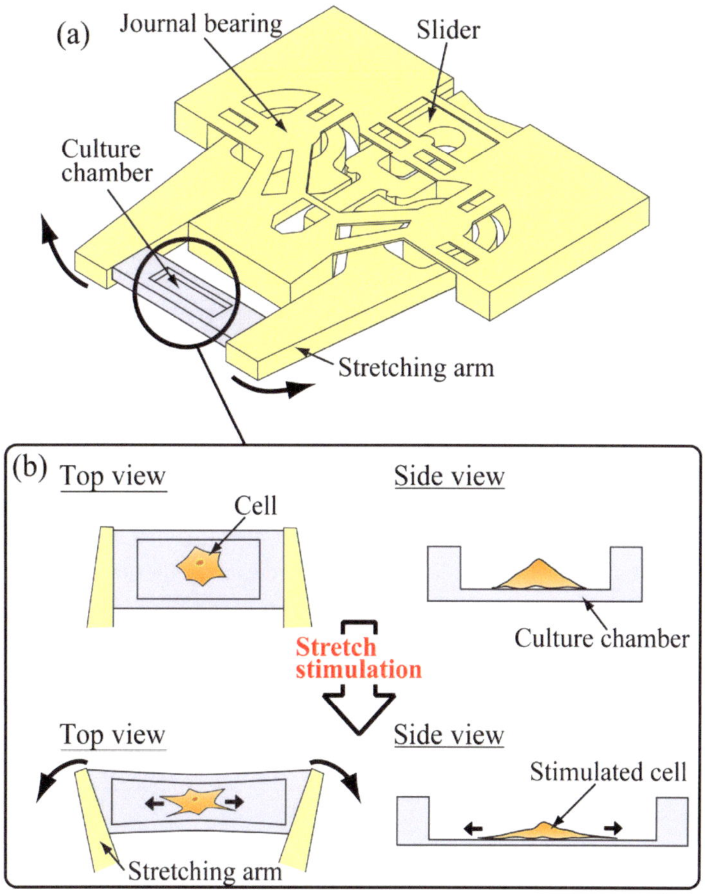

Fig. 11. Schematic of a fabricated mechanical stimulation micro device.

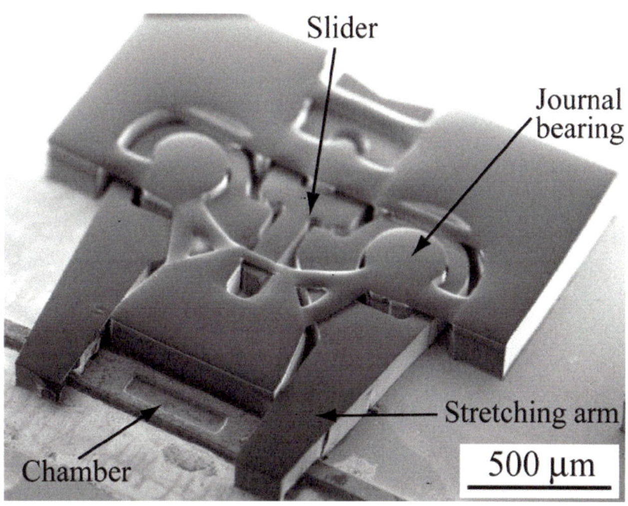

Fig. 12. SEM photograph of the fabricated mechanical stimulation micro device.

3.2 Device fabrication

The fabrication process of the device consists of two processes. One is the micromolding of silicone elastomer (PDMS) to fabricate the microchamber. The other is the patterning of thick photoresist to fabricate the link mechanism. The microchamber is made of transparent PDMS enable the observation using the inverted microscope. Although PDMS is generally used in the experiment of applying stretching deformation as a mechanical stimulus to cells (Costa et al., 2002), its chemical stability makes it difficult to shape by a microfabrication technique such as etching. Therefore, we adopted micromolding to fabricate the microchamber.

The fabrication process is shown in Fig. 13, and an outline of the process is described below. In the first step of the fabrication process of the microchamber, an original model of the microchamber for molding is prepared. The photoresist (SU-8, Kayaku MicroChem Co., Ltd) is spin-coated to 10 μm thickness (Fig. 13(a, b)), exposed and developed to pattern the stretching substrate (Fig. 13(c)). A second layer of SU-8 with 50 μm thickness is spin-coated onto the first layer (Fig. 13(d)), exposed and developed to pattern the support frame (Fig. 13(e)). By these two steps, an original model of the microchamber is obtained. In the next step, following the fabrication of the original model, the fluorine polymer is sprayed onto the original model to form very thin layer as mold-releasing agents (Fig. 13(f)). PDMS (KE-106, Shin-etsu Silicone) is casted on the original model to obtain a mold transcribed with the shape of the original model (Fig. 13(g)). The obtained mold is again sprayed with fluorine polymer, and punched to form the gate for molding (Fig. 13(h, i)). Finally, the microchamber made of PDMS is molded by using the obtained mold. The link mechanism is fabricated by the multilayer SU-8-based MEMS process (Foulds, I.G. & Parameswaran, M, 2006). This fabrication process includes multiple exposures to obtain movable three-dimensional microstructures.

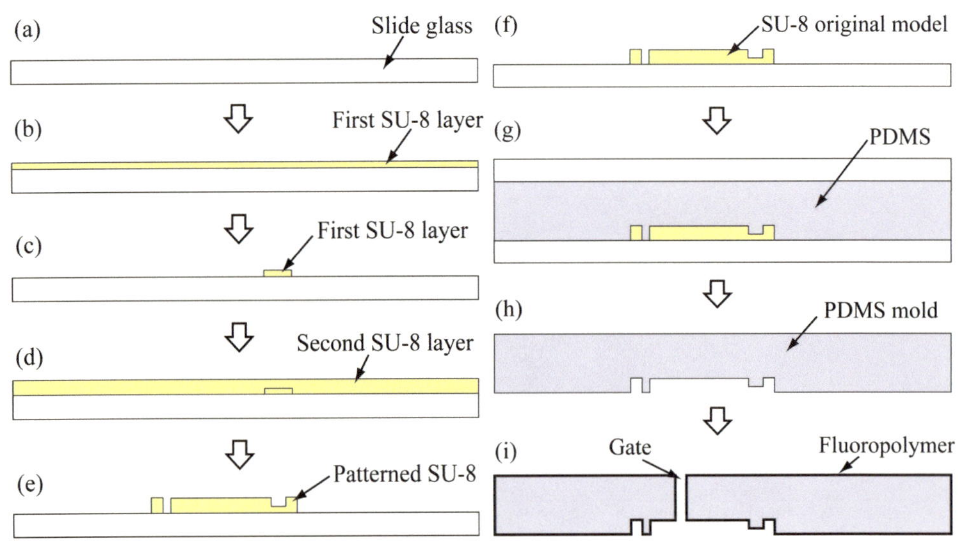

Fig. 13. Fabrication process of the original model and the micromold for the fabricated microchamber.

The fabrication process chart is shown in Fig. 14, and an outline of the process is described below. First, Ge is sputtered onto the glass coverslip and patterned as the sacrificial layer by which the microchamber (Fig. 14(j)), stretching arms and slider part are rendered movable. The PDMS microchamber is molded on the Ge-patterned coverslip (Fig. 14(l-n)). The first layer of SU-8 is spin-coated to 100 μm thickness (Fig. 14(o)), and exposed using the photomask of the link mechanism pattern (Fig. 14(p). In addition, without development, the second layer of SU-8 is spin-coated to 50 μm thickness on the first layer (Fig. 14(q)). The second exposure is applied to pattern the axis of the journal bearing (Fig. 14(r)). Finally, the surface exposure technique is applied to fabricate the stopper of the journal bearing (Fig. 14(s)). After the curing and the development of the entire device structure (Fig. 14(t)), the Ge sacrificial layer is removed and the link mechanism is completed (Fig. 14(u)).

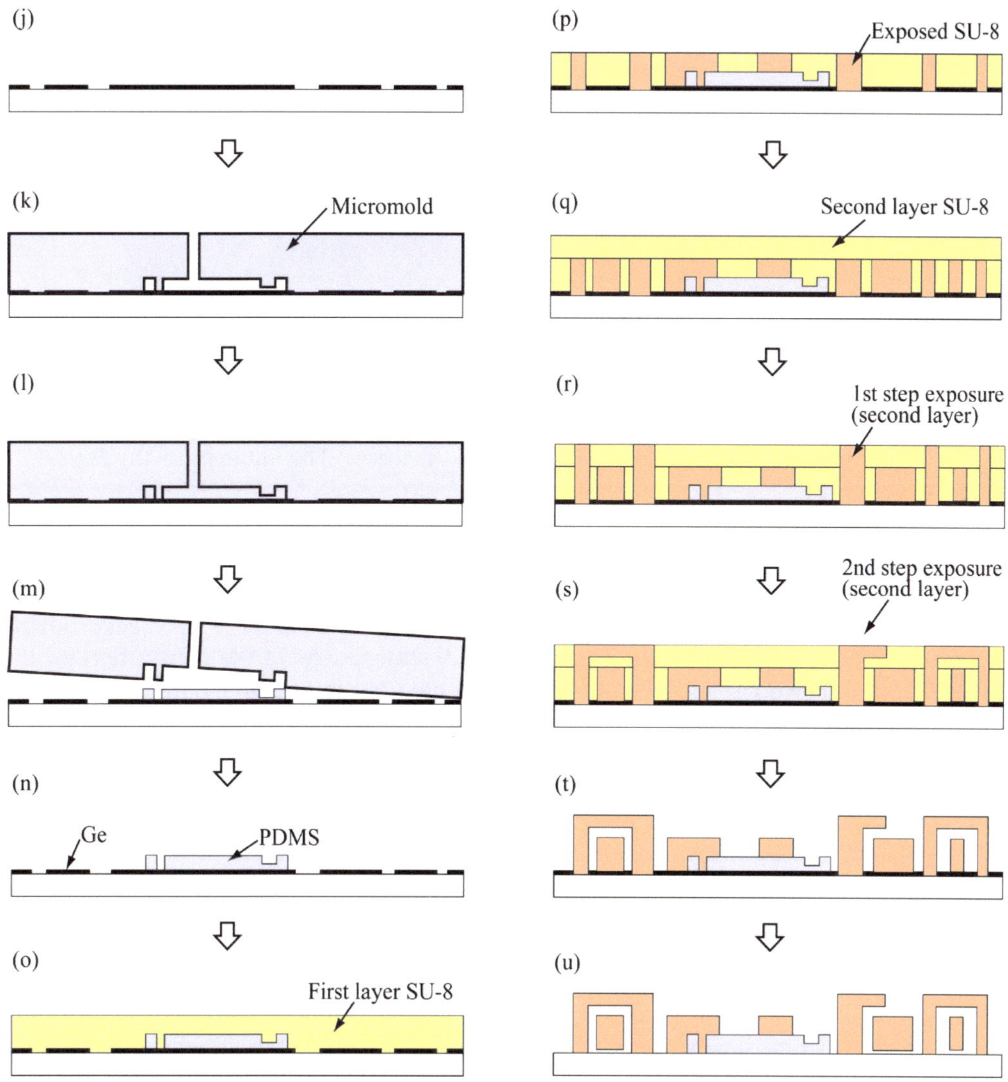

Fig. 14. Fabrication process of the microlink mechanism for mechanical stimulation device.

3.3 Operation test of mechanical stimulation device

The fabricated device on the glass coverslip was immersed in DI (deionized) water and tested. Figure 15 shows the image during the operation test using an inverted phase-contrast microscope (Olympus Co., CKX-41). Figure 15(a) shows the initial state of the device. Figure 15(b) shows the state after the slider was pushed by tweezers and the microchamber was stretched from both ends in the directions to the right and lift in the figure. It was shown that the fabricated device was actually able to work under observation using the inverted optical microscope.

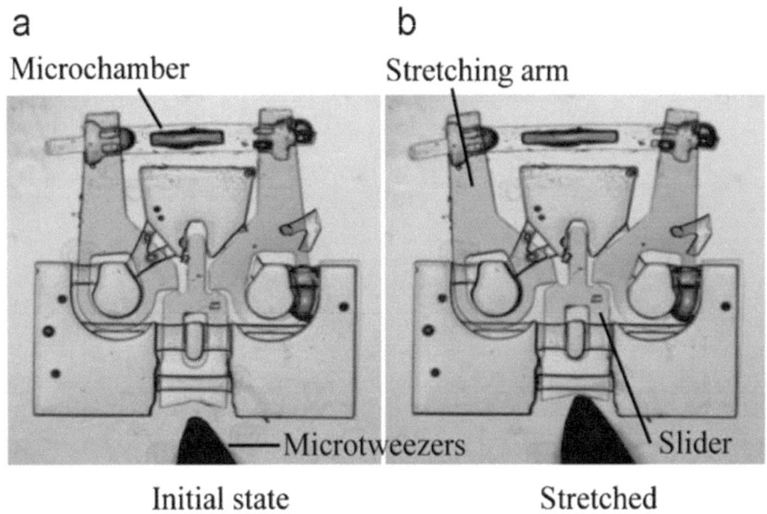

Fig. 15. Operating image of mechanical stimulation device. (a) The initial state. (b) The stretched state.

3.4 Cell stretching test by the mechanical stimulation device

We carried out the biocompatibility test by cell culture on the fabricated mechanical stimulation device. The cells were incubated using D-MEM with 10 % FBS (Fetal Bovine Serum), and in 37 °C, humidified 95 % air-5 % CO_2 atmosphere. In the preparation for the test, cultured cells were seeded into the dish with the built-in cell-stretching microdevices, and incubated for 8h. After the preincubation, fluorescent indictor dye Fluo 3 was loaded to the cell as the observation marker by incubating the cell in the opti-MEM containing 12 μM Fluo 3-AM (Dojindo) for 30 min. After loading the indicator dye, the cells were rinsed twice with PBS (phosphate buffered saline), and used for the test in normal culture medium. The epifluorescent inverted microscope was used for observation with a x 60 oil immersion objective lens.

Figure 16 shows the time lapse image of the stimulated single cell cultured on the chamber. For the sequential stretching operation, Fig. 16(b) shows an image immediately before the operation where we define t = 0.0 s. Cells are located slightly above the center in the figure. Two particles slightly below the center are dust particles of fluorescence dye. Figure 16(c) shows an image immediately after the stretching operation, t = 0.1 s. Stretching operation was continued to t = 0.7 s (Fig. 16(f)) and the amount of maximum nominal tensile strain in stretching axis was roughly estimated as 13 % by measuring the displacement of dust

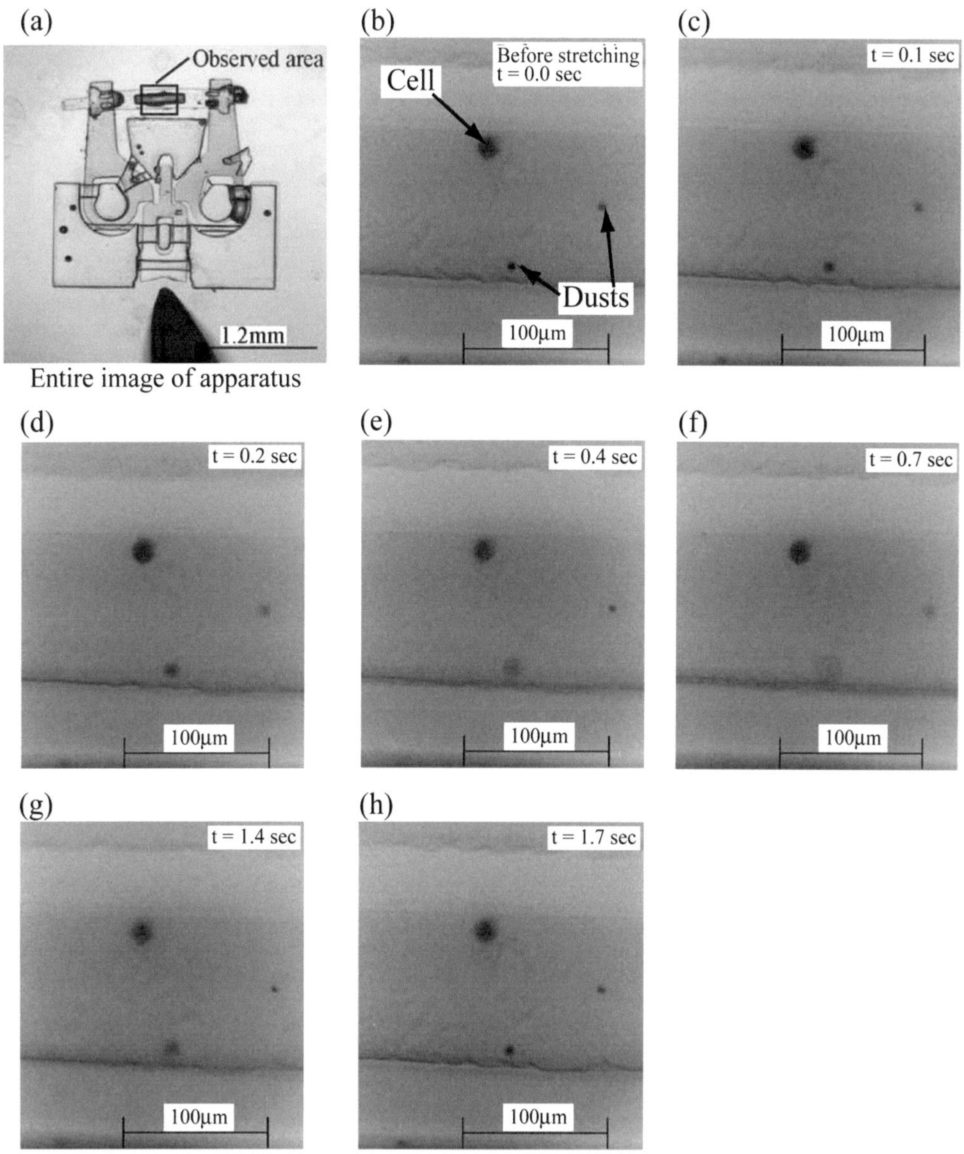

Fig. 16. Sequential time lapse images of a single cell uniaxially stretched using mechanical stimulation micro device. Dark gray indicates higher fluorescent intensity.

particles. Immediately after the maximum stretching, the stretching operation was stopped, and the microchamber returned to the initial state at t = 1.7 s (Fig. 16(h)). As a result, the cell successfully adhered to the stretched substrate and received the stretching stimulation in the microchamber. This result indicates that the fabricated mechanical stimulation device is biocompatible and able to apply dynamic mechanical stimulus to a cell. Also, the observed cell stayed in the field of view, indicating that this device can reduce the rigid displacement of the cell during the stretching operation. Therefore, this device can be used in the observation experiments of reaction to a mechanical stimulus of a cell such as the alteration of cellular morphology and cell differentiation induction.

4. Conclusions

This paper demonstrated that two micro devices for dynamic cell differentiation induction. First, we demonstrated that a chemical stimulation micro device consisting of nano-hole array for chemical release and a hydrophobic passive microvalve for its release control is effective in controlling NGF concentration that is required to control stimulation to a cell. Release of chemical solution such as culture medium could be controlled precisely by opening and closing the microvalve because the microvalve was placed very close to the nano-hole array. Furthermore, we succeeded in cell differentiation guidance by controlling NGF release from nano-hole array.

On the other hand, we evaluated the performance of the mechanical stimulation micro device consisting of the culture chamber, the stretching arms, the journal bearings and the slider. Mechanical stimulation to a cell can be controlled by regulating of the chamber contraction with the slider operation. We succeeded in observation of the single cell reaction behavior stimulated by stretching. This result indicated this device can induce the cell differentiation by stimulation control based on cellular reaction.

These devices are able to evaluate the response and morphology transformation of pheochromocytoma based on the chemical/mechanical stimulation. Also, these results suggest that the fabricated two devices can dynamically induce the stem cell differentiation by controlling chemical and mechanical stimulation.

5. Acknowledgment

This work was partly supported by a fund from the MEXT (Ministry of Education, Culture, Sports, Science and Technology) via the Grant-in-Aid for Scientific Research (B) and for Young Scientists (B), and also by the "Development of Nanotechnology and Materials for Innovative Utilizations of Biological Functions" Project of the Ministry of Agriculture, Forestry and Fisheries of Japan.

6. References

Lanza, R. & Rosenthal, N. (2004). *Scientific American,* Nature America Inc., ISBN 0036-8733, America

Meyer, J.-U.; Schuttler, M.; Thielecke, H. & Stieglitz, T. (2000). Biomedical Microdevices for Neural Interfaces. *Proceedings of the 1st Annual international IEEE-EMBS Special Topic*

Conference on Microtechnologies in Medicine and Biology, ISBN 0-7803-6603-4, Lyon, France, August 2000

Takeuchi, S. & Shimoyama, I. (1999). Three Dimensional SMA Microelectrodes with Cliipping Structure for Insect Neural Recording. *Technical Digest of the twelfth IEEE International Conference on Micro Electro Mechanical Systems*, ISBN 0-7803-5194-0, Orlando, FL, January 1999

Nakashima, Y.; Hata, S. & Yasuda, T. (2010). Blood Plasma Separation and Extraction from a Minute Amount of Blood Using Dielectrophoretic and Capillary Forces. *Sensors and Actuators B: Chemical*, No. 145, (2010), pp. 561-569, ISSN 9025-4005

Nakashima, Y. & Yasuda, T. (2009). Parallel Preparation of Microliquid Mixtures Using Wettability Gradient and Electrowetting, *Proceedings of the Micro Total Analysis Systems Symposium 2009*, ISSN 1556-5904, Jeju, Korea, November 2009

Chen, D.F.; Du, H., & Li, W.H. (2007). Bioparticle Separation and Manipulation Using Dielectrophoresis. *Sensors and Actuators A: Phisical*, 133, (2007), pp. 329-334, ISSN 9024-4247

Taff, B.M. & Voldman, J. (2005). A scalable addressable posirive-dielectrophoretic cellsorting array. *Analytical Chemistry*, 77, 24, (2005), pp. 7976-7983, ISSN 1520-6882

Choi, S. & Park, J.K. (2005). Microfluidic System for Dielectrophoretic Separation Based on a Trapezoidal Electrode Array. *Lab on a Chip*, 5, (2005), pp. 1161-1167, ISSN 1473-0189

Doh, I. & Cho, Y.H. (2005). A Continuous Cell Separation Chip Using Hydrodynamic Dielectrophoresis Process. *Sensors and Actuators A: Phisical*, 121, (2005), pp. 59-65, ISSN 9024-4247

Nakashima, Y. & Yasuda, T. (2002). Fabrication of a Microfluidic Device for Axonal Guidance. *Journal of Robotics and Mechatoronics*, Vol. 17, No. 2, (April 2005), pp. 158-163, ISSN 0915-3942

Yun, K.-S.; Lee, S.-I.; Lee, G.M., & Yoon, E. (2002). Design and fabrication of micro/nano-fluidic chip performing single-cell positioning and nanoliter drug injection for single-cell analysis. *Proceedings of the Micro Total Analysis Systems Symposium 2002*, ISSN 1556-5904, Nara, Japan, November 2002

Lee, N.Y.; Yamada, M., & Seki, M. (2002). Improved sample injection method adapting hydrophobic passive valve systems for microfluidic devices. *Proceedings of the Micro Total Analysis Systems Symposium 2002*, ISSN 1556-5904, Nara, Japan, November 2002

Nakashima, Y. & Yasuda, T. (2007). Cell Differentiation Guidance Using Chemical Stimulation Controlled by a Microfluidic Device. *Sensors and Actuators A: Physical*, 139, (June 2007), pp. 252-258, ISSN 0924-4247

Sato, K.; Kamada, S. & Minami, K. (2010). Development of Microstretching Device to Evaluate Cell Membrane Strain Field Around Sensing Point of Mechanical Stimulation. *International Journal of Mechanical Sciences*, 52, (2010), pp. 251-256, ISSN 0020-7403

Costa, K.D.; Hucker W.J., & Yin, FC-P. (2002). Buckling of Actin Stress Fibers: a New Wrinkkle in The Cytoskeletal Tapestry. *Cell Motility and the Cytoskeleton*, 52, (2002), pp. 266-274, ISSN 1097-0169

Foulds, I.G. & Parameswaran, M. (2006). A Planar Self-sacrificial Multilayer SU-8-based MEMS Process Utilizing a UV-blocking Layer for the Creation of Freely Moving Parts. *Journal of Micromechanics and Microengineering*, 16, (2006), pp. 2109-2115, ISSN 0960-1317

Part 3

Pathophysiology 3. Signaling Pathways

5

Phospholipase A_2 and Signaling Pathways in Pheochromocytoma PC12 Cells

Alexey Osipov and Yuri Utkin
Shemyakin-Ovchinnikov Institute of Bioorganic Chemistry, Russian Academy of Sciences
Russia

1. Introduction

Phospholipases A_2 (PLA2s) (phosphatidylcholine 2-acylhydrolases, EC 3.1.1.4) are ubiquitous lipolytic enzymes. PLA2s are widely spread in nature; they have been found in many organisms including mammals, reptiles, invertebrates, plants, fungi, ameba, bacteria, and viruses as well as in snake and bee venom. The PLA2s include five distinct types of enzymes: the secreted PLA2s (sPLA2), the cytosolic PLA2s, the Ca^{2+} independent PLA2s, the platelet-activating factor acetylhydrolases, and the lysosomal PLA2s (Schaloske & Dennis 2006); a new type, so-called adipose-specific PLA2, has been described recently (Duncan et al., 2008). PLA2s form a numerous protein superfamily, which is divided into 15 groups and many subgroups basing on their amino acid sequences, molecular masses, origin, number of disulphide bonds, Ca^{2+}-dependence and so on.

"Conventional" sPLA2s belonging to groups I/II/V/X are closely related, 13–19-kDa secreted enzymes with a highly conserved Ca^{2+}-binding loop, a catalytic site with a His–Asp dyad, six absolutely conserved disulfide bonds and up to two additional unique disulfide bonds, which contribute to the high degree of stability of these enzymes (Murakami et al., 2011). They require calcium at a level of extracellular environment for the lipolytic activity. For examples, PLA2s of group I are monomers of 13-15 kDa with 7 disulfide bridges. Among these, there are PLA2s of group IA found in Elapidae snake venom and those of group IB found mostly in mammalian pancreas. Group II of PLA2s comprises 6 sub-groups: sub-groups IIA and IIB are typical for Viperidae snake venom whereas sub-groups IIC-IIF are typical for mammalian tissues. Group III comprises sPLA2s from mammals, lizards, and bee venom (Schaloske & Dennis 2006).

Cytosolic PLA2s have no apparent homology to sPLA2s and differ from the latter in molecular mass, which is in the range from 60 to 115 kDa, stability to thiol reagents and requirement in calcium at a cytosolic level which, in contrast to the sPLA2s, is required rather for translocation of the enzyme to intracellular membranes than for catalysis. Cytosolic PLA2s utilize the Asp-Ser catalytic dyad; phosphorylation of the Ser residue enhances lipolytic activity (Schaloske & Dennis 2006). These PLA2s are found only in vertebrates (Murakami et al., 2011).

Ca^{2+}-independent PLA2s are referred to so-called patatin-like phospholipase domain-containing lipases (Murakami et al., 2011). Like cytosolic PLA2, they utilize a serine for catalysis (Schaloske & Dennis 2006).

The main effect of PLA2 is the hydrolysis of the sn-2 position of glycerophospholipids to release fatty acid (as a rule, unsaturated one, especially arachidonic acid, 20:4 *n*–6) and 2-lysophospholipids. The down-stream enzymes of arachidonate methabolism are cyclooxygenases and lipoxygenases (COXs and LOXs). Arachidonic acid is a key precursor of various eicosanoids including prostaglandins, thromboxanes and leukotrienes with their own biological activities. In addition to (or along with) lipolytic activity, PLA2s may exert a broad spectrum of biological effects. So, they may impact different cell functions as well as display pro-inflammatory, platelet-activating, cytotoxic and other stress response-inducing properties (see reviews (Boyanovsky & Webb, 2009; Lambeau & Gelb, 2008)) and even anti-bacterial action (mainly of group IIA, (Buckland & Wilton, 2000; Nevalainen et al., ,2008)). sPLA2s from venoms may also possess anticoagulant activity, presynaptic neurotoxicity, myo- and cytotoxicity. The main biological activities of PLA2s from different groups along with their effects on PC12 cells are summarized in table 1. Some of these diverse effects depend on the enzymatic activity while others do not. In certain cases, e.g., affecting blood coagulation, some of sPLA2s need to hydrolyze phospholipids to gain an anti-coagulant effect while others show the anti-coagulant activity *per se*, without such hydrolysis (Kini, 2005). The non-enzymatic effects may involve different mechanisms, for example, protein-protein interactions (Hanasaki, 2004; Lambeau & Lazdunsky, 1999; Valentin & Lambeau, 2000), which will be discussed below.

None of known PLA2s exerts all variety of the above biological effects. To explain snake venom sPLA2 functional specificity, Kini and Evans (Kini, 2005; Kini & Evans, 1989) have proposed a so-called "target model". According to this model, surface of a target cell or tissue have a "target site" ("target protein") which is recognized by a complementary "pharmacological site" in the PLA2 molecule. The affinity between PLA2s and target proteins lies in the nanomolar range, whereas the affinity between PLA2s and phospholipids covers the micromolar range. Such a difference may explain why the interaction of venom PLA2 with target protein governs the pharmacological specificity (Kini, 2005). The "pharmacological site" is independent of, but sometimes overlapping with, the active enzymatic site. Of course, neighboring phospholipids may also contribute to the interaction (Kini, 2005).

A variety of membrane and soluble proteins strongly bind $sPLA_2s$, suggesting that the $sPLA_2$ enzymes could also function as high affinity ligands (Hanasaki, 2004; Valentin & Lambeau, 2000). Most of the binding data have been accumulated with venom $sPLA_2s$ and group IB and IIA mammalian $sPLA_2s$. In general, venom $sPLA_2s$ have been shown to bind to membrane and soluble mammalian proteins of the C-type lectin superfamily (M-type $sPLA_2$ receptor and lung surfactant proteins), to N-type receptors, to pentraxin and reticulocalbin proteins, and to factor Xa (see review (Valentin & Lambeau, 2000)). M-type PLA2 receptor has been found in muscle first (therefore - M) and then identified in other organs; the PLA2 binding to this receptor is calcium-insensitive. N-type PLA2 receptor has been found in brain (N - neuronal); more recently N-type-like PLA2 receptors have been found in other organs. The PLA2 binding to this receptor is calcium-dependent. These receptors selectively bind certain sPLA2s with picomolar affinity. So, bee venom PLA2 binds to N-type and M-type receptors with IC_{50} of 80 pM and >0.3 μM, respectively. The affinity of OS1, a PLA2 from taipan snake venom, for these two receptors is quite different: 34 pM for M-type and 1.5 μM for N-type, while OS2 from taipan binds these receptors with almost equal affinity (6 and 10 pM for M- and N-type, respectively) (Lambeau & Lazdunski, 1999). Hence, some additional mechanism(s) besides phospholipide hydrolysis should be considered in

PLA2 group	Distribution	Main activity(s)	Effect(s) on PC12
IA	Elapidae snake venom	Acute toxicity, cytotoxicity; platelet aggregation, anticoagulant.	Differentiation, cytotoxicity.
IB	Pancreatic secretions, lung, liver, spleen, kidney, brain	Digestion of dietary PLs; antibacterial; eicosanoid formation; cell contraction, proliferation, migration, pyknosis.	
	Elapidae snake venom		Differentiation
IIA	Acute phase serum, intestinal mucosa, lacrimal gland cells, prostatic epithelial cells	Inflammation, acute phase protein; antibacterial; atherogenic; anti-tumor or pro-tumorigenic; cell proliferation, migration, apoptosis; exocytosis and neurotransmitter release.	Apoptosis; exocytosis and neurotransmitter release.
	Viperidae snake venom	Acute toxicity, cytotoxicity, miotoxicity, neurotoxicity; platelet aggregation, anticoagulant.	Differentiation; cytotoxicity; exocytosis and neurotransmitter release (blockage at internal application).
III	Kidney, heart, liver, skeletal muscle, epididymus, placenta, leukocytes	Sperm maturation; pro-tumorigenic; antiviral.	Differentiation; cell survival.
	Bee venom	Inflammation; cytotoxicity, pyknosis; antibacterial.	Differentiation, cytotoxicity.
V	Heart, eye, lung, pancreas, macrophages, neutrophils, mastocytes	Antibacterial, antifungal, antiviral; atherogenic; eicosanoid generation; phagocytosis.	Differentiation.
X	Gastrointestinal tract, stomach, lung, testis, spleen, thymus, neutrophils, macrophages	Antibacterial, antiviral, atherogenic, pro-tumorigenic.	Differentiation.
XIII	Bacteria/fungi	Modulation of host inflammatory response.	Differentiation.
Cytosolic PLA2s	Kidney, brain, heart, spleen, thyroid	Inflammation, anaphylaxis; ulceration; acute lung injury, brain injury; parturition; nociception; junction proteins through or from the Golgi.	Apoptosis, hypoxic or ischemic cell death; partition in exocytosis.
Ca-independent PLA2s	Different cell types	Cell activation, proliferation, migration, or apoptosis, pro-tumorigenic; secretion; control of energy metabolism in adipocytes.	Apoptosis, hypoxic or ischemic cell death; regulation of exocytosis.

Table 1. The main biological activities of PLA2s and their effects on PC12 cells. The table includes only those PLA2 groups that have been shown to act on/in PC12 cells. The data have been compiled mainly from (Boyanovsky & Webb, 2009; Farooqui, 2009; Murakami et al., 2011; Nakashima et al., 2003; Schaloske & Dennis 2006).

signaling pathways in which PLA2s take part. For example, it has been suggested that "neuronal" effects of sPLA2s derived from animal venoms may be mediated by their specific binding to N-type receptor on neuronal membranes (Hanasaki, 2004). It should be noted, that to date there is no direct evidence on presence of a sPLA2 receptor in PC12 cells (neither of C-lectin-like nor of any other type).

There is a lot of data that PLA2s may display neurotoxic properties. They may affect also some important neuronal functions, such as neurotransmitter release and neuronal survival as well as neuritogenesis. Thus, there is no coincidence that PLA2s are found in nerve growth cones in PC12 cells. We do not intend to discuss here all the effects of PLA2 on various types of neuronal cells as it has already done in overall by others (for instance, see respective chapters in (Farooqui, 2009) and other reviews). In accordance with the topic of the present book, we shall consider in details the PLA2 effects mainly on PC12 cell line.

2. PLA2 and neurite outgrowth in PC12 cells

PC12 cell line has been derived from rat pheochromocytoma which is a tumor of neuronal origin. This cell line serves sometimes as a convenient model for studying some "neuronal" effects of different compounds. It is known for many years that PC12 cells are also capable to exhibit neurite outgrowth upon appropriate external stimulation. This process may be evoked by application of different biochemical agents: polypeptides (e.g., neurotrophins: nerve growth factor (NGF) or fibroblast growth factors, and some neuropeptides of secretin superfamily (e.g., PACAP) (Ravni et al., 2006; Vaudry et al., 2002)), cAMP, which seems to be a messenger of the latters (Gerdin & Eiden, 2007), and its certain derivatives (Gunning et al., 1981), sialoglycosides (Ledden et al., 1990) and sialic acid precursors (Kontou et al., 2009), lectins (Wu et al., 2004), some phospholipide metabolites (discussed below), calcium ions (by membrane depolarization), etc. Biochemical pathways converting signals from such diverse molecules to the neurite outgrowth may be either very different or almost identical, may overlap, or supplement, or amplify each other. For example, the differentiation pathways in PC12 are summarized in (Eiden et al., 2011). In all cases, the neurite outgrowth in PC12 is accompanied by shifting from a chromaffin cell-like phenotype to a neurite-bearing sympathetic neuron-like phenotype and results in termination of proliferation. The sum of these events is considered as an indicator of cell differentiation (Nakashima et al., 2004), the process opposed to malignant growth. Thus, PC12 is an excellent model to study at a cellular level the neuronal differentiation and antiproliferative effects of different compounds. In this paper we undertake the first attempt to systematize the data about effects of PLA2s on PC12 and to consider the possible mechanism(s) involved in these processes. However, we should say that PC12 cells in non-differentiated and differentiated forms have been documented to display at certain circumstances their own endogenous secretory, cytosolic, and calcium-independent PLA2 activity.

There is a number of papers discussing a role of activation of intracellular phospoholipase C or phospholipase D in NGF-induced PC12 differentiation (as well as in some other cellular events). The effects of these enzymes will not be considered in details in the present paper.

At the same time, increased activity of endogenous PLA2 has been found in nerve growth cones in differentiating PC12 and much of this PLA2 activity has been shown to be calcium-independent and secretory rather than cytosolic (Martin, 1998) or solely secretory (Ferrini et al., 2010). One cannot assert, however, that the activation of endogenous PLA2 is indeed an initial cause of neuritogenesis.

Along with the above mentioned substances, exogenous sPLA2s derived from different sources have been also found to induce the neurite outgrowth as well as produce some other effects in PC12 cells. Such a "neuritogenic" property has been already reported for sPLA2s of groups IA and IB from cobra venom (Makarova et al., 2006; Osipov et al., 2010), IIA from viper venom (Makarova et al., 2006), III from bee venom (Nakashima et al., 2003) and from human neuronal cells (Masuda et al., 2008), V from mouse (Nakashima et al., 2003), X from mouse (Nakashima et al., 2003) and human (Ikeno et al., 2005; Masuda et al., 2005), as well as XIII from bacteria and fungi (Nakashima et al., 2003). According to the early report (Hanada et al., 1996), fungal PLA2 p15 promotes only NGF-induced neuritogenesis but itself alone fails to induce neurite outgrowth in PC12; however, under some conditions p15 can displays neuritogenic properties (Wakatsuki et al, 1999). The concentrations at which sPLA2s begin to exert the neuritogenic effect are quite different. So, sPLA2 from bee venom being the most active among studied sPLA2s induces neurite outgrowth at concentration as low as 0.1 nM. sPLA2 of group XIII is effective starting from 1 nM (Nakashima et al., 2003), and snake venom sPLA2s of groups IA, IB, and IIA are effective at concentrations of 1-10 μM (Makarova et al., 2006; Osipov et al., 2010). Not all of sPLA2s can induce neuritogenesis: for example, mammalian sPLA2s of groups I and II are unable to produce this effect (Nakashima et al., 2003), while PLA2s of these groups from snake venom and mammalian PLA2s of groups V and X are effective in inducing neurite outgrowth .

It is assumed now that neurite outgrowth stimulated by PLA2s in PC12 cells is induced by the products of phospholipids hydrolysis and/or by their metabolites. Numerous data argue for this assumption. For instance, lysophosphatidylcholine (LPC) but not other lysophospholipids or arachidonic acid has been shown to promote the neurite outgrowth (Ikeno et al., 2005; Masuda et al., 2008). Overproduction or suppression of G2A, a G-protein-coupled receptor involved in LPC signaling, results in the enhancement or reduction, respectively, of neuritogenesis induced by sPLA2 treatment (Ikeno et al., 2005). LPC (either exogenously added or generated in situ by sPLA2-catalysed phosphatidyl choline hydrolysis) acts through an L-type Ca^{2+} channel-dependent mechanism. No synergistic enhancement of both sPLA2-promoted and LPC-induced neuritogenesis is produced by the co-addition of 100 μM arachidonic acid (Nakashima et al., 2003). Another way for LPC signaling is an activation of cytosolic phospholipase D2 which is involved in the regulation of depolarization-induced PC12 cell differentiation through activation of tyrosine kinases Pyk2(Y881) and ERK (extracellular signal-regulated kinase). However, action of different phospholipid products on PC12 is multilateral and dependent on certain extra factors. For example, similarly to PLA2 docosahexaenoic acid (22:6 *n*-3) is present in neurite growth cones. This acid decreases time-course activity of cytosolic PLA2 (Martin, 1998) and attenuates (Kim et al., 2001) or accelerates (Schonfeld et al., 2007) apoptotic death in PC12 cells. On the other hand arachidonic acid suppresses neurite outgrowth induced by nerve growth factor (Ikemoto et al., 1997) and also may be both anti-apoptotic (Kim et al., 2001) and pro-apoptotic at deprivation of NGF and serum (Atsumi et al., 1997) in PC12 (see also section 4). The above mentioned phospholipase D2 hydrolyzes the lysophospholipids with the formation of lysophosphatidic acid, which enhances cell proliferation. In differentiated PC12 cells lysophosphatidic acid provokes a rapid withdrawal of neurites (Moolenaar et al., 2004).

The direct relationship between the PLA2 enzymatic and differentiating activities may not be always evident. A number of papers (Ikeno et al., 2005; Nakashima et al., 2003; Nakashima et al., 2004) argues that anti-proliferative activity of PLA2s in PC12 is directly related to enzymatic activity. It has been suggested (Ikeno et al., 2005) that the binding of bee venom sPLA2 to the putative neuronal N-type receptor (see above) unlikely to be involved in PLA2-induced neurite outgrowth in PC12 cells. However, the data of (Nakashima et al., 2003) are contradictory to these conclusions: it has been shown that in PC12 cells catalytically inactive mutants of sPLA2s from groups V and X in which the active site His has been replaced by Ala exhibit neuritogenic activity that is only two times smaller than that of the native forms. Therefore, the His residue in the active site only promotes but does not determine the neuritogenic activity of sPLA2s in PC12. Another example showing that phospholipid hydrolysis is not the single requirement for the neuritogenic activity is a sPLA2 from Egyptian cobra venom: it possesses very weak enzymatic activity but induces neurite outgrowth in PC12 even more efficiently than cobra venom sPLA2 with strong enzymatic activity (Osipov et al., 2010).

Tumor cells of definite types can change their shape and stop proliferation being separated from a substrate. In whole, this is true for PC12 cells too. The possible role of extracellular matrix in the PLA2-induced neuritogenesis becomes evident from the following data. When PC12 cells are grown on polyethyleneimine used as a plate coat, fungal PLA2 p15 is unable to induce neurites but can only enhance the effect of NGF (Hanada et al., 1996). On the other hand it is known that collagen is the most effective purified extracellular matrix component supporting PC12 cell adhesion and NGF-induced neurite outgrowth. If the PC12 cells are grown on collagen-coated surface, p15 alone induces neurite outgrowth at concentration as low as 1 nM and does not require the addition of NGF for this effect (Wakatsuki et al, 1999). Moreover, the effect of p15 is faster than that of NGF: small neurites appear after 6 h of p15 treatment versus 24 h in the case of NGF (Wakatsuki et al, 1999).

3. Interdependent action of PLA2 and other agents

PC12 cells express sodium, potassium, and calcium ion channels and receptors for a lot of different ligands (grouth factors, neurotransmitters, adenosine and so on); effects of all these membrane proteins are in strong interdependence. At the first place, there are receptors for growth factors. There are two classes of receptors for NGF on cell surface: high affinity TrkA, a receptor tyrosine kinase which is highly specific for NGF, and a low affinity p75 neurotrophin receptor which binds all members of the neurotrophin family with a similar affinity (Skaper, 2008). Activation of p75 results in apoptosis of PC12 cells while activation of TrkA results in their differentiation. There is one intriguing and so far unexplained observation that NGF and several other agents are mitogens for normal chromaffin cells, but are anti-proliferative agents and induce neuronal differentiation of PC12 cells (Tischler et al., 2004). It should be mentioned that NGF induces an activation of the Na^+, K^+-pump in PC12 cells and increases sodium influx. Moreover, some researchers have seen small changes in cAMP level and in calcium currents evoked by NGF while others have not.

In PC12 cells NGF increases mRNA level for cytosolic PLA2 after treatment for 4h and cytosolic PLA2 protein level at 24h after beginning of treatment via the ERK1/2, p38 MAPK and PKC pathways (Akiyama et al, 2004). The following data support synergism in PLA2 and NGF action (Masuda et al., 2008). Adenoviral expression of human sPLA2 of group III (PLA2-III) in PC12 cells or dorsal root ganglion explants facilitates neurite outgrowth, whereas expression of a catalytically inactive PLA2-III mutant or use of PLA2-III-directed small interfering RNA (siRNA) reduces NGF-induced neuritogenesis. The results of the experiment with siRNA suggest that endogenous sPLA2-III profoundly affects neuritogenesis of PC12 cells. PLA2-III also suppresses neuronal death induced by NGF deprivation. In principle, this work (Masuda et al., 2008) demonstrates that the effects of NGF and PLA2 are different, however they complement each other. Thus, the overexpression of PLA2 replaces NGF, while NGF is not effective if PLA2 is switch off.

The data on blockage of PC12 differentiation evoked either by NGF or by PLA2 indicate that different pathways are involved in effects of these two agents. Thus, tyrosine kinase inhibitor K-252a blocks differentiation induced by NGF. Unlike NGF, neuritogenesis induced by sPLA2s is insensitive to K-252a. In contrary, inhibition of L-type calcium channel or depletion of extracellular calcium, which are ineffective in blocking NGF-induced neuritogenesis, may inhibit sPLA2-induced neurite outgrowth (Wakatsuki et al., 1999).

On the other hand, NGF activates not only tyrosine kinase cascade but also phospholipases C and A_2 which in turn results in enhance of arachidonate release from the cell lipids (Tsukada et al., 1994). Phosphorylation *in vitro* and *in vivo* of cytosolic PLA2 by mitogen-activated protein kinase at Ser505 increases its intrinsic enzyme activity several fold (Lin et al., 1993). After NGF treatment, the PLA2 activity in the PC12 cell lysate increases 4-fold on the third day (Ferrini et al., 2010) and during 7 days increases approximately 1.5-fold (Matsuzawa et al., 1996) i.e., effects of NGF and PLA2 on PC12 cells are mediated by different but somehow related mechanism(s). NGF changes the subcellular localization of group IIa endogenous sPLA2 in PC12 cells. In untreated cells, this PLA2 is mainly cytosolic and mitochondrial in localization. As soon as 6 h after NGF stimulation, it is no longer associated with mitochondria being found diffusely in the cytoplasm and associated with the plasma membrane as well as in growth cones at specific membrane domains. After 24 h, IIA PLA2 is detected within neurites and, at longer periods, the enzyme is mostly localized at neurite tips of neuron-like differentiated cells, as determined by confocal laser immunofluorescence microscopy analysis using anti-rat group IIA PLA2 monoclonal antibody (Ferrini et al., 2010). After treatment with NGF under identical conditions, group V PLA2 retains its cytoplasmic and nuclear localization and is scarcely present within neurites and neurite tips.

PC12 cells themselves comprise enzymes for synthesis of both catecholamines and acetylcholine. At the same time they bear acetylcholine receptors of both nicotinic and muscarinic types; stimulation of the formers results in the release of catecholamines while stimulation of the latter results in calcium influx and phosphoinositide hydrolysis (Fujita et al., 1989).

Calcium ion influx through voltage-gated channels triggers a variety of cellular events leading to neurite outgrowth via the concerted action of various calcium-binding proteins. Calcium influx mediates induction of gene expression in response to membrane depolarization. In PC12 cells, L-type channels are the primary carrier of voltage-sensitive calcium currents and have been shown to be required for sPLA2-induced neuritogenesis (Nakashima et al., 2003). The calcium signal transduction pathway promoting neurite outgrowth causes the rapid activation of protein tyrosine kinases, which include MEK1 and Src. They, in turn, further activate Ras (small guanine nucleotide-binding protein) and MAP kinase. A set of stimuli evokes the calcium influx; simultaneously cytosolic PLA2s are activated which results in release of arachidonic acid and other products of phospholipid hydrolysis. Interestingly, such a calcium-dependent activation of the cytosolic PLA2 does not need the extracellular calcium, and calcium from intracellular stores would be enough. Activation of an exogenous sPLA2 (either applied externally or expressed in PC12 cells) requires an influx of extracellular calcium. Thus, sub-millimolar and sub-micromolar Ca^{2+}

concentrations are necessary for activation of secretory and cytosolic PLA2s, respectively (Matsuzawa et al., 1996). Similarly to calcium as well as NGF pathways (Rusanescu et al., 1995; Vaudry et al., 2002), the sPLA2-induced neuritogenesis in PC12 involves the activation of Src and Ras proteins and is accompanied by the activation of MAPK cascade (Wakatsuki et al., 1999). The existing data indicate that PLA2, NGF, and calcium ions can act independently but synergistically in PC12 cells. However, as all of them activate the Ras/MAPK cascade, it is reasonable to suggest that their signaling pathways partially overlap.

Endogenous PLA2s in PC12 can be activated by different damaging agents (cyanides, reactive oxygen species, some cytolysins, etc.) that results in release arachidonic acid and its metabolites. Arachidonic acid being released by diacylglycerol hydrolysis promotes the opening of L- and/or N-type calcium channels that may lead to neurite outgrowth. Furthermore, the direct addition of arachidonic acid to the culture medium stimulates neurite outgrowth when PC12 cells grow on a fibroblast monolayer. However, arachidonic acid does not increase the steady-state calcium levels in neuronal growth cones (Nakashima et al., 2003, as cited in Walsh & Doherty, 1997). From existing data it is still not obvious, whether one of the activation pathway induced by either PLA2 or calcium channels begins first and then evokes other one.

Besides NGF receptor, PC12 express also two classes of epidermal growth factor receptors (activation of which in contrast to NGF receptor results in enhancement of PC12 proliferation, (Vaudry et al., 2002)) and receptors for fibroblast growth factor. To our knowledge, there are no data published on any cross-interaction of these receptors and PLA2.

Thus, PLA2s induce different cellular responses via very complex biochemical pathways in which PLA2s themselves or products of their enzymatic activity interact with various substances. These interactions are shown in a simplified form in Fig.1.

4. PLA2 in apoptosis and cytotoxicity

There are a lot of reports on the cytotoxic property of sPLA2s. This property is mostly attributable to PLA2s from animal venom. Concerning cytotoxicity of PLA2 in respect to PC12, it should be mentioned that sPLA2s from bee venom at concentrations higher than 10 nM (Nakashima et al., 2003), and from cobra and viper venoms at concentrations 10 μM and higher (Makarova et al., 2006) are toxic for these cells (i.e., induce the necrotic changes). Thus, cytotoxicity of many venom PLA2s attenuates strongly their "therapeutic" potential for differentiating action (section 2). However, non-cytotoxic sPLA2s (e.g., mammalian sPLA2s of groups V, X, and fungal/bacterial XIII (Nakashima et al., 2003), as well as a non-cytotoxic variant of venom sPLA2 (Osipov et al., 2010)) still preserve this potential and can be regarded antiproliferative agents.

Some toxic agents (for examples, reactive oxygen species produced by cyanides (Kanthasamy et al., 1997), by hydrogen peroxide (Akiyama et al., 2005), and so on) require cytosolic PLA2 activity for their damaging action.

A mechanism of endogenous sPLA2 cytotoxicity remains unknown yet. Sometimes, researchers assign it to enzymatic activity and to released arachidonate. In several cases such correlation may be traced, indeed. For instances, arachidonic acid itself being added to PC12 in concentrations above 10 μM kills the cells within 1-2 hours and does not require extracellular Ca^{2+} for the toxic effect. The removal of extracellular Ca^{2+} dramatically

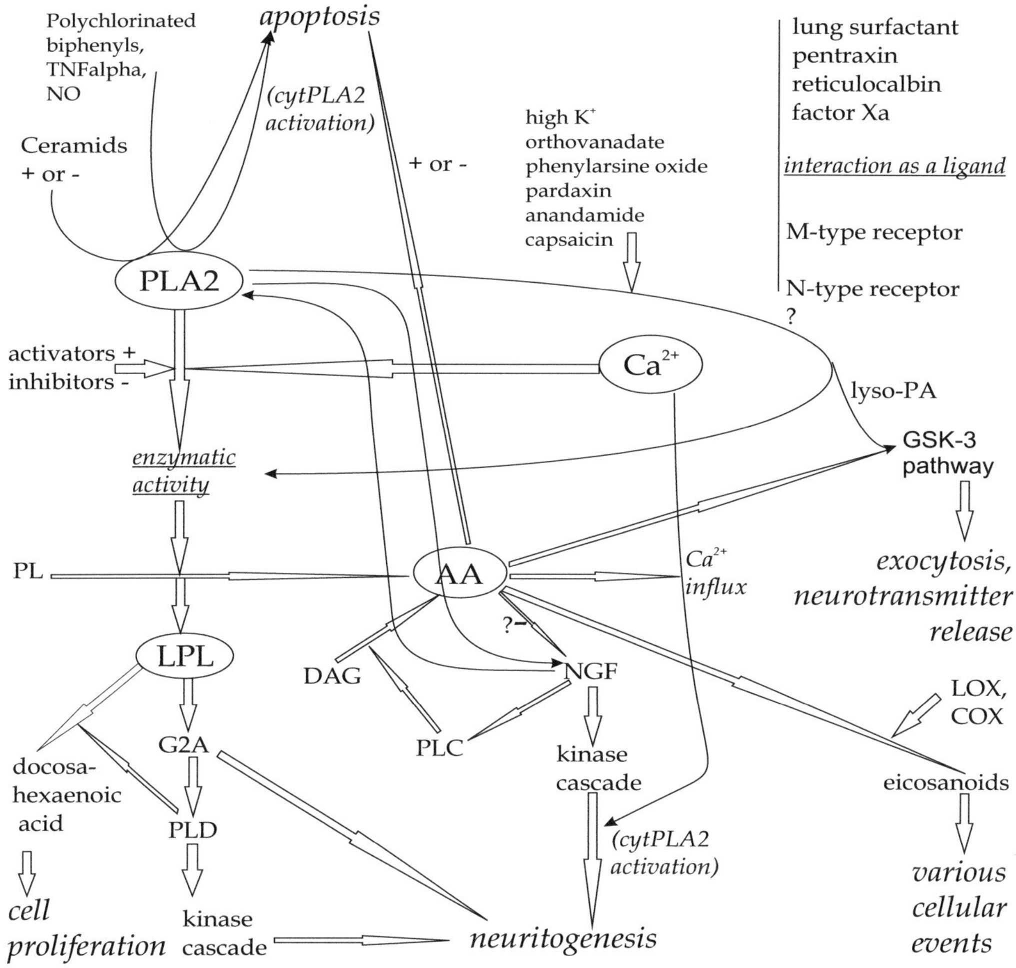

Fig. 1. Scheme of PLA2 interactions with the various substances mentioned in the text. The key players are in the ellipses; the processes considered are italicized. Inhibiting effects are indicated by minus, stimulating effects - by plus. DAG is diacylglycerol, PL is a phospholipide, lyso-PA is lyso-phosphatidic acid, and PLC and PLD are phospholipases C and D, respectively.

accelerates the acute cell death (Doroshenko & Doroshenko, 2004). Cytolysins impair ionic permeability of cell membrane, leading to cell death. Several different cytolysins have been tested on PC12 cells and found to enhance PLA2 activity as well as levels both of arachidonic acid and certain its metabolites (Raya et al., 1993). Peroxynitrite-dependent release of arachidonate by sPLA2 is supposed to be casually linked to peroxynitrite-dependent induction of DNA cleavage and toxicity (Guidarelli et al., 2000). However, there are enough reports (including cited in this paper) on PLA2s which possess high enzymatic activity and devoid of apparent cytotoxicity. Moreover, several papers describe the role of arachidonate in programmed cell death (apoptosis) but not in acute cytotoxicity.

PC12 may undergo apoptotic cell death under some stimuli (for example, under NGF deprivation or by activating p75 NGF receptor). PLA2s have been shown to take part in this process and extracellular Ca^{2+}-dependent release of arachidonic acid by sPLA2 is considered to mediate their action (Atsumi et al., 1997). Association of sPLA2 with cell surface proteoglycan, which has been shown to be a prerequisite for endogenous sPLA2-dependent arachidonic acid release from the plasma membranes of live cells, is not essential for sPLA2-mediated hydrolysis of apoptotic cell membranes. The authors give evidences that the apoptotic cell membrane is a potential target for extracellular type II sPLA2 (Atsumi et al., 1997). Arachidonic acid, a signaling lipid potentially associated with tumor necrosis factor receptor-I signal cascade, induces apoptosis in PC12 cells through inhibition of both protein kinase C zeta and nuclear factor kappaB activity. Apoptosis induced by arachidonate cannot be prevented by NGF (Macdonald et al., 1999).

Controversially, arachidonic acid has been reported to prevent neuronal apoptosis during serum starvation and COX and LOX do not participate in this process (Kim et al., 2001). Another research group has reported that arachidonic acid shows normal survival of NGF-differentiated PC12 whereas stearic acid and palmitic acid induce apoptotic cell death (Ulloth et al., 2003).

Several compounds have been reported to induce apoptosis in PC12 cells and in many cases PLA2 activity appears to be essential. For examples, short- and long-chain sphingosines are mediators of many cellular events including apoptosis in both naïve and NGF-differentiated PC12 (Posse de Chaves, 2006). C2-Ceramide (N-acetyl-D-erythro-sphingosine) alone stimulates arachidonic acid release and enhances the ionomycin-induced release. In contract, some sphingosines show an opposite effect and directly inhibite cytosolic phospholipase A2alpha activity (Nakamura et al., 2004). Nitric oxide can induce apoptosis. Nitric oxide is involved in the regulation of cytosolic PLA2, its phosphorylation and activity, arachidonic acid release and as consequence in up-regulation of expression and activity of COXs and LOXs; blockage of their activity may rescue cell death (Pytlowany et al., 2008). In neuronal PC12 cells, TNF-alpha induces moderate apoptosis. Application of TNF-alpha to the PC12 cells results in p38 MAPK phosphorylation and activation. Phosphorylation of p38 MAPK is regulated by cytosolic PLA2, which produces arachidonic acid. The results present one possible mechanism for enhancing the neuronal cell death by arachidonate through the regulation of p38 MAPK. However, how arachidonate attenuates the phosphorylation of p38 MAPK is unknown (Park et al., 2002).

Ortho-substituted polychlorinated biphenyls induce apoptosis in PC12. These compounds evoke PLA2-mediated Ca^{2+} influx. However, in the presence of extracellular Ca^{2+}, PLA2 activation is inhibited by neither an extracellular nor an intracellular Ca^{2+} chelator but is depressed by inhibitors of calcium-independent PLA2 (Shin et al., 2002).

Along apoptosis, PC12 cells may undergo hypoxic or ischemic caspase-independent cell death characterized by nuclear shrinkage (pyknosis). This process comes with participation of calcium-independent PLA2 and, to a lesser extension, cytosolic PLA2. Interestingly, bee venom PLA2 and porcine pancreatic sPLA2 also can cause nuclear shrinkage in another cell type. Neither arachidonate nor other fatty acids (stearic, linoleic, palmitic, and oleic acids) induces the shrinkage suggesting that PLA2 induces nuclear shrinkage itself and that its metabolites are ineffective (Shinzawa & Tsujimoto, 2003).

Thus, calcium-independent PLA2 seems to play an important role in programmed cell death in PC12 that is consistent with the data on participation of group VIA calcium-independent PLA2 in apoptosis in cell types other than PC12 (Balsinde et al., 2006; Lei et al., 2010). Cytosolic PLA2 also seems to participate in apoptosis.

Nevertheless, it is not quite understood yet why a PLA2 activity in PC12 results in cell necrosis in several cases, in apoptosis in some cases, and in differentiation in other.

5. Exocytosis and secretion in PC12 cells and PLA2

As PC12 cells are tumor scions of neuroendocrine chromaffin cells, it is relevant to mention the PLA2 action on catecholamine secretion in the chromaffin cells. Pre-synaptic neurotoxic snake venom sPLA2, taipoxin, enhances exocytosis in bovine chromaffin cells in response to depolarizing stimuli. It entries into the cytosol, that is already detectable after 5 min and is independent on extracellular calcium, i.e., the toxin does not use calcium-dependent endocytosis to reach the chromaffin cell cytoplasm. After 1 h, a large portion of the toxin has redistributed to the plasma membrane and fragmentation of the F-actin cytoskeleton is observed; an increased number of events of granule fusion takes place during the initial phase of secretion with an enhancement of the initial rate of release, and after 1 day, cell death becomes evident (Neco et al., 2003). Authors (Giner et al., 2007) propose mechanism according to which, in neuroendocrine chromaffin cells, neurotoxic sPLA2s bind to surface membrane receptors and hydrolyze phospholipids that results in release of lysophosphatidic acid among other products. This product activates intracellular pathways involving the glycogen synthase kinase 3 (GSK-3), an important modulator of many physiological processes, such as neurodevelopment, the cell cycle, apoptosis and oncogenesis (either as a suppressor or as a promoter) (Mishra, 2010), causing cytoskeleton alterations with neurite retraction. Alterations in actin cytoskeleton result in the loosening of the peripheral cortex barrier thus facilitating the access of secretory granules to the release sites of the plasmalemma (Giner et al., 2007).

There is a lot of indications on the participation of PLA2s in exocytosis in PC12. On the one hand, PLA2 may participate in regulation of cell secretion; on the other hand, sPLA2 itself may be released by exocytosis. sPLA2 of group II is involved in the regulation of neurotransmitter secretion by PC12 cells. The neurotransmitters released from PC12 cells by PLA2 are catecholamines and acetylcholine. PLA2 seems to be involved also in the degranulation process in neuronal cells and itself may influence exocytosis in PC12 cells.

External application of group IIA sPLA2 (purified crotoxin subunit B from snake venom or purified human synovial sPLA2) causes an immediate increase in exocytosis and neurotransmitter release in PC12 cells, detected by carbon fiber electrodes placed near the cells, or by changes in membrane capacitance of the cells. There is an indication that the effect of sPLA2 is dependent on calcium and sPLA2 enzymatic activity (Wei et al., 2003). When type II sPLA2 purified from rat platelets is added to NGF-treated PC12 cells, there is a dose-dependent release of both noradrenaline and dopamine, reaching a maximum release of ~10% at 20-40 μg/ml sPLA2 after 10-30 min of incubation. Release of dopamine by exogenous sPLA2 is dependent on extracellular calcium. Interestingly, thielocin A1, a type II sPLA2-specific inhibitor, or neutralizing antibody against type II sPLA2 suppress noradrenaline release in a dose-dependent manner. These results indicate that endogenous sPLA2 may be involved in catecholamine secretion from PC12 cells. The concentration of exogenous type II sPLA2 required for catecholamine secretion from PC12 cells is higher than that which can be released from activated PC12 cells (Matsuzawa et al., 1996). Secretion of dopamine from PC12 cells that is stimulated by glutamate is suppressed by type II sPLA2 inhibitors. Exogenous type II sPLA2 added alone directly elicites release of dopamine from PC12 cells (Kudo et al., 1996). Because the antibody could not pass through the plasma membrane without permeabilization, it is likely that sPLA2 might act from outside the cells, becoming accessible to the antibody after cell activation. This is supported by the fact that exogenously added sPLA2 directly elicites dopamine release from PC12 cells in an extracellular Ca^{2+}-dependent manner (Matsuzawa et al., 1996).

In contrast to external application, internal application of sPLA2 to PC12 cells produces blockade of neurotransmitter release (Wei et al., 2003).

It was suggested (Matsuzawa et al., 1996) that arachidonic acid metabolism elicited by neurotransmitters or by depolarization, which mobilizes intracellular Ca^{2+}, is more likely to be regulated by cytosolic PLA2. However, the authors do not rule out the possibility for hydrolysis of membrane phospholipids by sPLA2 to liberate arachidonic acid, which leads to catecholamine secretion. Arachidonic acid may be released from PC12 cells in response to different stimuli. Thus, it is released from undifferentiated PC12 under NGF action (Tsukada et al., 1994). PLA2 also promotes release of arachidonate from NGF-differentiated PC12 cells which are stimulated, for examples, by staphylococcal alpha-toxin at subcytotoxic concentrations (Fink et al., 1989), peroxynitrite (by activation of endogenous sPLA2) (Guidarelli et al., 2000), high K^+ or via direct stimulation of phospholipide hydrolysis by mastoparan, a tetradecapeptide PLA2 activator from bee venom (Ray et al., 1999). Several other compounds including orthovanadate, phenylarsine oxide, pardaxin, anandamide and capsaicin have been reported to induce the arachidonate releasing by PLA2 from PC12 treated with NGF, with subsequent prostaglandin F2alpha formation. Orthovanadate activates cytosolic PLA2 to release arachidonate, stimulates tyrosine phosphorylation in proteins and enhances Ca^{2+}-induced noradrenaline release (Mori et al., 2001). Phenylarsine oxide acts probably via activation of endogenous secretory PLA2; it may act synergistically with exogenous sPLA2 from bee venom (Ohsawa et al., 2002). Pardaxin, an α-helical cytolysin from the fish *Pardachirus marmoratus*, aggregates in the plasma membrane to form ionic channels, followed by calcium influx. By this way it activates calcium-dependent PLA2, but it also can activate calcium-independent PLA2 in PC12 (Abu-Raya et al., 1998). Anandamide and capsaicin stimulate arachidonic acid release even in the absence of extracellular calcium. The effects of anandamide and capsaicin are inhibited by PLA2 inhibitors, but not by an antagonist for vanilloid VR1 receptor (Someya et al., 2002). Exocytosis in PC12 may be evoked also by lysophosphatidylinositol, another product of phospholipid hydrolysis by sPLA2 (Ma et al., 2010).

Arachidonate release is associated with acetylcholine release in NGF-differentiated PC12 cells. Botulinum neurotoxin type A (BoTx) inhibits this process. K^+-stimulated acetylcholine release is also totally inhibited by pretreatment of cells with BoTx (2 nM). Inclusion of exogenous arachidonate, or the PLA2 activator melittin, or bee venom sPLA2 itself prevents the effect of BoTx (Ray et al., 1993). Treatment of differentiated PC12 cells with mastoparan and high (80 mM) K^+ induces acetylcholine exocytosis. The acetylcholine release depends upon Ca^{2+} influx via the N-type voltage-sensitive Ca^{2+} channels. The release is followed by a rise in intracellular free Ca^{2+} concentration; the increased Ca^{2+} activates PLA2 and, thereby, increases the arachidonate level (Ray et al., 1999). BoTx cleaves SNAP-25, a conserved synaptosomal protein essential for vesicle fusion and docking during neuroexocytosis. Blockage of SNAP-25 function by the antisense oligonucleotides has shown that the neuroexocytosis involving PLA2 activity proceeds without participation of this protein. Moreover, mastoparan prevents the neurotoxic effect of BoTx through induction PLA2 activity that seems not to involve SNAP-25 pathway (Ray et al., 1999).

Differentiated PC12 cells, being stimulated with carbamylcholine, potassium, or glutamate, release sPLA2 into the medium. Thus, sPLA2 of group II is released in response to stimulation by neurotransmitters or depolarization. sPLA2 is released from neuronally differentiated PC12 cells upon stimulation by carbamylcholine via acetylcholine receptors or by high K^+ via voltage-dependent Ca^{2+} channels through membrane depolarization (Matsuzawa et al., 1996). When NGF-treated PC12 cells are activated with glutamate, approximately 40% of their group II sPLA2 is released into the extracellular medium. Glutamate-stimulated secretion of dopamine from PC12 cells is PLA2-dependent, as it is suppressed by group II sPLA2 inhibitors (Kudo et al., 1996).
As after activation of PC12 cells by carbamylcholine, the time courses of noradrenaline and sPLA2 release are not parallel (the release of noradrenaline reaches a plateau at 10 min and that of sPLA2 at 15 min), sPLA2 and catecholamine may be stored in different secretory granules (Matsuzawa et al., 1996).
A recent report has appeared concerning a role of calcium independent PLA2 in exocytosis and mitochondrial function in PC12: inhibition of this type of PLA2 results in excessive exocytosis through increased oxidative damage (or failure to repair such damage) and defects in mitochondrial function (Ma et al., 2011).
It is still unclear, however, whether the relation between neurotransmitter signaling/release and the effects of PLA2 plays a significant role in other discussed processes including the PC12 differentiation.

6. Conclusion

In general, PLA2s are involved in different signaling pathways in PC12 cells. Various types of PLA2s and even groups within types may exert diverse effects on the cells. Most of them in one or another way are now associated with phospholipid products. One should note, however, that it would not be correct to attribute such diversity of effects to enzymatic activity of PLA2 only. Understanding the mechanisms involved in PC12 differentiation induced by PLA2s may results in development of new drugs inhibiting tumor cell proliferation.
As it has been discussed in this paper, PLA2 enzymes manifest a number of very diverse biological properties. At the same time, PC12 cell line is a valuable model for study of different signaling mechanisms. The effects of PLA2s on PC12 cells are quite complex and multifaceted. Several striking findings have already been made upon investigation of these effects and one can expect further exciting findings in this area.

7. Acknowledgment

The work on this paper has been supported by Russian Foundation for Basic Research (grants # 09-04-01061 and 10-04-00708).

8. References

Abu-Raya, S., Bloch-Shilderman, E., Shohami, E., Trembovler, V., Shai, Y., Weidenfeld, J., Yedgar, S., Gutman, Y. & Lazarovici, P. (1998). Pardaxin, a new pharmacological tool to stimulate the arachidonic acid cascade in PC12 cells. *The Journal of pharmacology and experimental therapeutics*, Vol.287, No.3, (December 1998), pp. 889-896, ISSN 0022-3565

Akiyama, N., Hatori, Y., Takashiro, Y., Hirabayashi, T., Saito, T. & Murayama, T. (2004). Nerve growth factor-induced up-regulation of cytosolic phospholipase A2alpha level in rat PC12 cells. *Neuroscience letters*, Vol. 365, No.3, (July 2004), pp. 218-222. ISSN 0304-3940

Akiyama, N., Shimma, N., Takashiro, Y., Hatori, Y., Hirabayashi, T., Horie, S., Saito, T. & Murayama, T. (2005). Decrease in cytosolic phospholipase A2alpha mRNA levels by reactive oxygen species via MAP kinase pathways in PC12 cells: effects of dopaminergic neurotoxins. *Cellular signalling*, Vol.17, No.5, (May 2005), pp. 597-604, ISSN 0898-6568

Atsumi, G., Murakami, M., Tajima, M., Shimbara, S., Hara, N. & Kudo, I. (1997). The perturbed membrane of cells undergoing apoptosis is susceptible to type II secretory phospholipase A2 to liberate arachidonic acid. *Biochimica et Biophysica Acta*, Vol.1349, No.1, (November 1997), pp. 43-54. ISSN 0006-3002

Balsinde, J., Pérez, R. & Balboa, M.A. (2006). Calcium-independent phospholipase A2 and apoptosis. *Biochimica et Biophysica Acta*, Vol.1761, No.11, (November 2006), pp. 1344-1350, ISSN 0006-3002

Boyanovsky, B.B. & Webb, N.R. (2009). Biology of secretory phospholipase A2. *Cardiovascular drugs and therapy*, Vol.23, No.1, (February 2009), pp 61-72, ISSN 0920-3206

Buckland, A.G. & Wilton, D.C. (2000). The antibacterial properties of secreted phospholipases A(2). *Biochimica et Biophysica Acta*, Vol.1488, No.1-2, (October 2000), pp. 71–82, ISSN 0006-3002

Doroshenko, N. & Doroshenko, P. (2004). Ca^{2+} influx is not involved in acute cytotoxicity of arachidonic acid. *Biochemical pharmacology*, Vol.67, No.5, (March 2004), pp. 903-909, ISSN: 0006-2952

Duncan, R.E., Sarkadi-Nagy, E., Jaworski, K., Ahmadian, M. & Sul, H.S. (2008). Identification and functional characterization of adipose-specific phospholipase A2 (AdPLA). *Journal of biological chemistry*, Vol.283, No.37, (September 2008), pp. 25428-25436, ISSN 0021-9258

Eiden, L., Lazarovici, P., Vaudry, D., Stork, P.J.S. & Samal, B. (no date) Differentiation Pathway in PC12 Cells. In: *Sci. Signal. Connections Map in the Database of Cell Signaling*, 20.07.2011, available at http://stke.sciencemag.org/cgi/cm/stkecm;CMP_8038

Farooqui, A.A. (2009). *Hot Topics in Neural Membrane Lipidology*. Springer Science+Business Media, LLC, ISBN 978-0-387-09692-6, New York, USA.

Ferrini, M., Nardicchi, V., Mannucci, R., Arcuri, C., Nicoletti, I., Donato, R. & Goracci, G. (2010). Effect of NGF on the subcellular localization of group IIA secretory phospholipase A(2) (GIIA) in PC12 cells: role in neuritogenesis. *Neurochemical research*, Vol.35, No.12, (December 2010), pp. 2168-2174, ISSN 0364-3190

Fink, D., Contreras, M.L., Lelkes, P.I. & Lazarovici, P. (1989). Staphylococcus aureus alpha-toxin activates phospholipases and induces a Ca^{2+} influx in PC12 cells. *Cellular signalling*, Vol.1, No.4, pp. 387-393, ISSN 0898-6568

Fujita, K., Lazarovici, P. & Guroff, G. (1989). Regulation of the differentiation of PC12 pheochromocytoma cells. *Environmental health perspectives*, Vol.80, (March 1989), pp. 127-142, ISSN 0091-6765

Gerdin, M.J. & Eiden, L.E. (April 2007). Regulation of PC12 cell differentiation by cAMP signaling to ERK independent of PKA: do all the connections add up? In: *Science's STKE: signal transduction knowledge environment*, 17.04.2007, ISSN 1525-8882, Available from http://stke.sciencemag.org/cgi/content/abstract/sigtrans;2007/382/pe15

Giner, D., López, I., Neco, P., Rossetto, O., Montecucco, C. & Gutiérrez, L.M. (2007). Glycogen synthase kinase 3 activation is essential for the snake phospholipase A2 neurotoxin-induced secretion in chromaffin cells. *The European journal of neuroscience*, Vol.25, No.8, (April 2007), pp. 2341-2348, ISSN 0953-816X

Guidarelli, A., Palomba, L. & Cantoni, O. (2000) Peroxynitrite-mediated release of arachidonic acid from PC12 cells. *British journal of pharmacology*, Vol.129, No.8, (April 2000), pp. 1539-1541, ISSN 0007-1188

Gunning, P. W, Letourneau, P. C., Landreth, G. E., & Shooter, E. M. (1981).The action of nerve growth factor and dibutyryl adenosine cyclic 3', 5'-monophosphate on rat pheochromocytoma reveals distinct stages in the mechanisms underlying neurite outgrowth. *The Journal of neuroscience*, Vol.1, No.10, (October 1981), pp. 1085-1095 ISSN 0270-6474

Hanada, T., Sato, T., Arioka, M., Uramoto, M. & Yamasaki, M. (1996). Purification and characterization of a 15 kDa protein (p15) produced by Helicosporium that exhibits distinct effects on neurite outgrowth from cortical neurons and PC12 cells. *Biochemical and biophysical research communications*, Vol.228, No.1, (November 1996), pp. 209-215, ISSN 0006-291X

Hanasaki, K. (2004). Mammalian Phospholipase A2: Phospholipase A2 Receptor. *Biological & pharmaceutical bulletin*, Vol.27, No.8, pp. 1165-1167, ISSN 0918-6158

Ikemoto, A., Kobayashi, T., Watanabe, S. & Okuyama, H. (1997). Membrane fatty acid modifications of PC12 cells by arachidonate or docosahexaenoate affect neurite outgrowth but not norepinephrine release. *Neurochemical research*, Vol.22, No.6, (June 1997), pp. 671-678, ISSN 0364-3190

Ikeno, Y., Konno, N., Cheon, S.H., Bolchi, A., Ottonello, S., Kitamoto, K., & Arioka, M. (2005) Secretory phospholipases A2 induce neurite outgrowth in PC12 cells through lysophosphatidylcholine generation and activation of G2A receptor. *Journal of biological chemistry*, Vol.280, No.30, (July 2005), pp. 28044-28052, ISSN 0021-9258

Kanthasamy, A.G., Ardelt, B., Malave, A., Mills, E.M., Powley, T.L., Borowitz, J.L. & Isom, G.E. (1997). Reactive oxygen species generated by cyanide mediate toxicity in rat pheochromocytoma cells. *Toxicology letters*, Vol.93, No.1, (September 1997), 47-54, ISSN 0378-4274

Kim, H.Y., Akbar, M. & Kim, K.Y. (2001). Inhibition of neuronal apoptosis by polyunsaturated fatty acids. *Journal of molecular neuroscience*, Vol.16, No.2-3, (April-June 2001), pp. 223-227; discussion 279-284, ISSN 0895-8696

Kini, R.M. (2005). Structure-function relationships and mechanism of anticoagulant phospholipase A2 enzymes from snake venoms. *Toxicon*, Vol.45, No.8, (June 2005), pp. 1147-1161, ISSN 0041-0101

Kini, R.M. & Evans, H.J. (1989). A model to explain the pharmacological effects of snake venom phospholipases A2. *Toxicon*, Vol.27, No.6, pp. 613-635, ISSN 0041-0101

Kontou, M., Weidemann, W., Bork, K. & Horstkorte, R. (2009). Beyond glycosylation: sialic acid precursors act as signaling molecules and are involved in cellular control of differentiation of PC12 cells. *Biological chemistry*, Vol.390, No.7, (July 2009), 575-579, ISSN 1431-6730

Kudo, I., Matsuzawa, A., Imai, K., Murakami, M., & Inoue, K. (1996). Function of type II phospholipase A2 in dopamine secretion by rat neuronal PC12 cells. *Journal of lipid mediators and cell signalling*, Vol.14, No.1-3, (September 1996), 25-31, ISSN 0929-7855

Lambeau, G. & Gelb, M.H. (2008). Biochemistry and physiology of mammalian secreted phospholipases A(2). *Annual review of biochemistry*, Vol.77, pp. 495–520, ISSN 0066-4154

Lambeau, G. & Lazdunski, M. (1999) Receptors for a growing family of secreted phospholipases A2. *Trends in pharmacological sciences*, Vol.20, No.4, (April 1999), pp. 162-170, ISSN 0165-6147

Ledeen, R.W., Wu, G., Cannella, M.S., Oderfeld-Nowak, B. & Cuello, A.C. (1990). Gangliosides as neurotrophic agents: studies on the mechanism of action. *Acta neurobiologiae experimentalis*, Vol.50, No.4-5, pp. 439-449, ISSN 0065-1400

Lei, X., Barbour, S.E. & Ramanadham, S. (2010). Group VIA Ca2+-independent phospholipase A2 (iPLA2beta) and its role in beta-cell programmed cell death. *Biochimie*, Vol.92, No.6, (June 2010), pp. 627-637, ISSN 0300-9084

Lin, L.L., Wartmann, M., Lin, A.Y., Knopf, J.L., Seth, A. & Davis, R.J. (1993) cPLA2 is phosphorylated and activated by MAP kinase. *Cell*, Vol.72, No.2, Jan pp. 269-278, ISSN 0092-8674

Ma, M.T., Yeo, J.F., Farooqui, A.A., Zhang, J., Chen, P. & Ong, W.Y. (2010). Differential effects of lysophospholipids on exocytosis in rat PC12 cells. *Journal of neural transmission*, Vol.117, No.3, (March 2010), pp. 301-308, ISSN 0300-9564

Ma, M.T., Yeo, J.F., Farooqui, A.A. & Ong, W.Y. (2011). Role of calcium independent phospholipase A2 in maintaining mitochondrial membrane potential and preventing excessive exocytosis in PC12 cells. *Neurochemical research*, Vol.36, No.2, (February 2011), pp. 347-354, ISSN 0364-3190

Macdonald, N.J., Perez-Polo, J.R., Bennett, A.D. & Taglialatela, G. (1999). NGF-resistant PC12 cell death induced by arachidonic acid is accompanied by a decrease of active PKC zeta and nuclear factor kappa B. *Journal of neuroscience research*, Vol.57, No.2, (July 1999), pp. 219-226, ISSN 0360-4012

Makarova, Y.V., Osipov, A.V., Tsetlin, V.I. & Utkin, Y.N. (2006). Influence of phospholipases A2 from snake venoms on survival and neurite outgrowth in pheochromocytoma cell line PC12. *Biochemistry (Moscow)*, Vol.71, No.6, (June 2006), pp. 678-684, ISSN: 0006-2979

Martin, R.E. (1998). Docosahexaenoic acid decreases phospholipase A2 activity in the neurites/nerve growth cones of PC12 cells. *Journal of neuroscience research*, Vol.54, No.6, (December 1998), pp. 805-813, ISSN 0360-4012

Masuda, S., Murakami, M., Takanezawa, Y., Aoki, J., Arai, H., Ishikawa, Y., Ishii, T., Arioka, M. & Kudo, I. (2005). Neuronal expression and neuritogenic action of group X secreted phospholipase A2. *Journal of biological chemistry*, Vol.280, No.24, (June 2005), pp. 23203-23214, ISSN 0364-3190

Masuda, S., Yamamoto, K., Hirabayashi, T., Ishikawa, Y., Ishii, T., Kudo, I. & Murakami, M. (2008). Human group III secreted phospholipase A2 promotes neuronal outgrowth and survival. *The Biochemical journal*, Vol.409, No.2, (January 2008), pp. 429-438. ISSN 0264-6021

Matsuzawa, A., Murakami, M., Atsumi, G., Imai, K., Prados, P., Inoue, K. & Kudo, I. (1996). Release of secretory phospholipase A2 from rat neuronal cells and its possible function in the regulation of catecholamine secretion. *The Biochemical journal*, Vol.318, No.Pt 2, (September 1996), pp. 701-709, ISSN 0264-6021

Mishra, R. (June 2010). Glycogen synthase kinase 3 beta: can it be a target for oral cancer. In: *Molecular Cancer*, 11.06.2010, Available from: http://www.molecular-cancer.com/content/9/1/144

Moolenaar, W.H., van Meeteren, L.A. & Giepmans, B.N. (2004). The ins and outs of lysophosphatidic acid signaling. *BioEssays: news and reviews in molecular, cellular and developmental biology*, Vol.26, No.8, pp. 870-881, ISSN 0265-9247

Mori, A., Yasuda, Y., Murayama, T. & Nomura, Y. (2001). Enhancement of arachidonic acid release and prostaglandin F(2alpha) formation by Na_3VO_4 in PC12 cells and GH3 cells. *European journal of pharmacology*, Vol.417, No.1-2, (April 2001), pp. 19-25, ISSN 0014-2999

Murakami, M., Taketomi, Y., Miki, Y., Sato, H., Hirabayashi, T. & Yamamoto, K. (2011). Recent progress in phospholipase A(2) research: From cells to animals to humans. *Progress in lipid research*, Vol.50, No.2, (April 2011), pp. 152-192, ISSN 0163-7827

Nakamura, H., Hirabayashi, T., Someya, A., Shimizu, M. & Murayama, T. (2004). Inhibition of arachidonic acid release and cytosolic phospholipase A2 alpha activity by D-erythro-sphingosine. *European journal of pharmacology*, Vol.484, No.1, (January 2004), pp. 9-17, ISSN 0014-2999

Nakashima, S., Ikeno, Y., Yokoyama, T., Kuwana, M., Bolchi, A., Ottonello, S., Kitamoto, K., Arioka, M. (2003). Secretory phospholipases A2 induce neurite outgrowth in PC12 cells. *The Biochemical journal*, Vol.376, No.Pt 3, (December 2003), pp. 655-666, ISSN 0264-6021

Nakashima, S., Kitamoto, K. & Arioka, M. (2004). The catalytic activity, but not receptor binding, of sPLA2s plays a critical role for neurite outgrowth induction in PC12 cells. *Brain research*, Vol.1015, No.1-2, (July 2004), pp. 207-211, ISSN: 0006-8993

Neco, P., Rossetto, O., Gil, A., Montecucco, C. & Gutiérrez, L.M. (2003). Taipoxin induces F-actin fragmentation and enhances release of catecholamines in bovine chromaffin cells. J Neurochem. *Journal of neurochemistry*, Vol.85, No.2, (April 2003), pp. 329-337, ISSN 0022-3042

Nevalainen, T.J., Graham, G.G. & Scott, K.F. (2008). Antibacterial actions of secreted phospholipases A2. Review. *Biochimica et Biophysica Acta*, Vol.1781, No.1-2, (January-February 2008), pp. 1-9, ISSN 0006-3002

Ohsawa, K., Mori, A., Horie, S., Saito, T., Okuma, Y., Nomura, Y. & Murayama, T. (2002). Arachidonic acid release and prostaglandin F2alpha formation induced by phenylarsine oxide in PC12 cells: possible involvement of secretory phospholipase A2 activity. *Biochemical pharmacology*, Vol.64, No.1, (July 2002), pp. 117-124, ISSN 0006-2952

Osipov, A.V., Filkin, S.Y., Makarova, Y.V., Tsetlin, V.I. & Utkin, Y.N. (2010). A new type of thrombin inhibitor, noncytotoxic phospholipase A2, from the Naja haje cobra venom. *Toxicon*, Vol.55, No.2-3, (February-March 2010), pp. 186-194, ISSN 0041-0101

Park, J.G., Yuk, Y., Rhim,H., Yi, S.Y. & Yoo, Y.S. (2002). Role of p38 MAPK in the regulation of apoptosis signaling induced by TNF-alpha in differentiated PC12 cells. *Journal of biochemistry and molecular biology*, Vol.35, No.3, (May 2002), pp. 267-272, ISSN 1225-8687

Pytlowany, M., Strosznajder, J.B., Jeśko, H., Cakała, M. & Strosznajder, R.P. (2008). Molecular mechanism of PC12 cell death evoked by sodium nitroprusside, a nitric oxide donor. *Acta biochimica Polonica*, Vol.55, No.2, pp. 339-347. ISSN 0001-527X

Ravni, A., Bourgault, S., Lebon, A., Chan, P., Galas, L., Fournier, A., Vaudry, H., Gonzalez, B., Eiden, L.E. & Vaudry, D. (2006). The neurotrophic effects of PACAP in PC12 cells: control by multiple transduction pathways. *Journal of neurochemistry*, Vol.98, No.2, (July 2006), pp. 321-329, ISSN 0022-3042

Ray, P., Berman, J.D., Middleton, W. & Brendle, J. (1993). Botulinum toxin inhibits arachidonic acid release associated with acetylcholine release from PC12 cells. *Journal of biological chemistry*, Vol.268, No.15, (May 1993), pp. 11057-11064, ISSN 0021-9258

Ray, P., Ishida, H., Millard, C.B., Petrali, J.P. & Ray, R. (1999). Phospholipaise A2 and arachidonic acid-mediated mechanism of neuroexocytosis: a possible target of botidinum neurotoxin A other then SNAP-25. *Journal of applied toxicology*, Vol.19, Suppl 1, (December 1999), pp. S27-28, ISSN 0260-437X

Raya, S.A., Trembovler, V., Shohami, E. & Lazarovici, P. (1993). Cytolysins increase intracellular calcium and induce eicosanoids release by pheochromocytoma PC12 cell cultures. *Natural toxins*, Vol.1, No.5, pp. 263-270, ISSN 1056-9014

Posse de Chaves, E.I. (2006). Sphingolipids in apoptosis, survival and regeneration in the nervous system. *Biochimica et Biophysica Acta*, Vol.1758, No.12, (December 2006), pp. 1995-2015, ISSN 0006-3002

Rusanescu, G., Qi, H., Thomas, S.M., Brugge, J.S. & Halegoua, S. (1995). Calcium influx induces neurite growth through a Src-Ras signaling cassette. *Neuron*, 15, No.6, (December 1995), pp. 1415-1425 ISSN 0896-6273

Schaloske, R.H. & Dennis, E.A. (2006). The phospholipase A2 superfamily and its group numbering system. *Biochimica et Biophysica Acta*, Vol.1761, No.11, (November 2006), pp. 1246-1259, ISSN 0006-3002

Shin, K.J., Chung, C., Hwang, Y.A., Kim, S.H., Han, M.S., Ryu, S.H. & Suh, P.G. (2002). Phospholipase A2-mediated Ca2+ influx by 2,2',4,6-tetrachlorobiphenyl in PC12 cells. *Toxicology and applied pharmacology*, Vol.178, No.1, (January 2002), pp. 37-43. ISSN 0041-008X

Shinzawa, K. & Tsujimoto, Y. (2003). PLA2 activity is required for nuclear shrinkage in caspase-independent cell death. *The Journal of cell biology*, Vol.163, No.6, (December 2003), pp. 1219-1230 ISSN 0021-9525

Schonfeld, E., Yasharel, I., Yavin, E. & Brand, A. (2007). Docosahexaenoic acid enhances iron uptake by modulating iron transporters and accelerates apoptotic death in PC12 cells. *Neurochemical research*, Vol.32, No.10, (October 2007), pp. 1673-84, ISSN 0364-3190

Skaper, S.D. (2008). The biology of neurotrophins, signalling pathways, and functional peptide mimetics of neurotrophins and their receptors. *CNS and neurological disorders drug targets*, Vol.7, No.1, (February 2008), pp. 46-62, ISSN 1871-5273

Someya, A., Horie, S. & Murayama, T. (2002). Arachidonic acid release and prostaglandin F(2alpha) formation induced by anandamide and capsaicin in PC12 cells. *European journal of pharmacology*, Vol.450, No.2, (August 2002), pp. 131-139, ISSN 0014-2999

Tischler, A.S., Powers, J.F. & Alroy, J. (2004). Animal models of pheochromocytoma. *Histology and histopathology*, Vol.19, No.3, (July 2004), pp. 883-95, ISSN 0213-3911

Tsukada, Y., Chiba, K., Yamazaki, M. & Mohri, T. (1994). Inhibition of the nerve growth factor-induced neurite outgrowth by specific tyrosine kinase and phospholipase inhibitors. *Biological & pharmaceutical bulletin*, Vol.17, No.3, (March 1994), pp. 370-375, ISSN 0918-6158

Ulloth, J.E., Casiano, C.A. & De Leon, M. (2003). Palmitic and stearic fatty acids induce caspase-dependent and -independent cell death in nerve growth factor differentiated PC12 cells, *Journal of neurochemistry*, Vol.84, No.4, (February 2003), pp. 655-668, ISSN 0022-3042

Valentin, E. & Lambeau, G. (2000) Increasing molecular diversity of secreted phospholipases A2 and their receptors and binding proteins. *Biochimica et Biophysica Acta* Vol.1488, No.1-2, (October 2000), pp. 59–70, ISSN 0006-3002

Vaudry, D., Stork, P.J., Lazarovici, P. & Eiden, L.E. (2002). Signaling pathways for PC12 cell differentiation: making the right connections. *Science*, Vol.296, No.5573, (May 2002), pp. 1648-1649, ISSN 0036-8075

Wakatsuki, S., Arioka, M., Dohmae, N., Takio, K., Yamasaki, M. & Kitamoto, K. (1999). Characterization of a novel fungal protein, p15, which induces neuronal differentiation of PC12 cells. *Journal of biochemistry*, Vol.126, No.6, (December 1999), pp. 1151-1160, ISSN 0021-924X

Wei, S., Ong, W.Y., Thwin, M.M., Fong, C.W., Farooqui, A.A., Gopalakrishnakone, P. & Hong W. (2003). Group IIA secretory phospholipase A2 stimulates exocytosis and neurotransmitter release in pheochromocytoma-12 cells and cultured rat hippocampal neurons. *Neuroscience,* Vol.121, No.4, pp. 891-898, ISSN: 0306-4522

Wu, Y., Sheng, W., Chen, L., Dong, H., Lee, V., Lu, F., Wong, C.S., Lu, W.Y. & Yang, B.B. (2004). Versican V1 isoform induces neuronal differentiation and promotes neurite outgrowth. *Molecular biology of the cell,* Vol.15, No.5, (May 2004), pp. 2093-2104, ISSN: 1059-1524

6

Programmed Cell Death Mechanisms and Pheocromocytomas: Recent Advances in PC12 Cells

Davide Cervia and Cristiana Perrotta
University of Tuscia and University of Milan
Italy

1. Introduction

The endocrine system is a network of endocrine glands and nerves throughout the body. Endocrine glands produce and release hormones that circulate around the body in the blood. Hormones keep an even balance of chemicals and fluid within the body, and help us respond to changes in the environment. The endocrine system is made up of several glands, including the adrenal glands.

1.1 The adrenal medulla and its hormones

There are two adrenal glands in our body that produce a number of vital hormones essential for survival. The adrenal glands, located at the superior poles of the two kidneys, are composed of two distinct layers, the adrenal cortex and the adrenal medulla. The outer adrenal cortex, which develops from the abdominal mesothelium, surrounding the medulla during embryogenesis, synthesizes and secretes the adrenocortical hormones, the mineralocorticoids and glucocorticoids, as well as the adrenogenic (sexual) hormones.

The adrenal medulla, which comprises the central 20% of the gland, originates from the neural crest, and does not become distinct and compact until the adrenal cortex atrophies during the first few weeks postnatally. The adrenal medulla is a modified sympathetic ganglion which secretes in the bloodstream the catecholamines epinephrine (adrenaline) and norepinephrine (noradrenaline) in response to sympathetic neural stimulation to the medullae. Depending on the physiological conditions, this secretion averages 80% epinephrine to 20% norepinephrine. Although dopamine is present in the adrenal and serves as a precursor for norepinephrine and epinephrine, minimal dopamine secretion occurs and the role of adrenal dopamine is not well understood.

Cells of the medulla are known as pheochromocytes or chromaffin cells, referring to the dark color produced by the polymerization of oxidized catecholamines when these cells are exposed to chromium salts. The early medulla also contains neuroblasts and developing sympathetic ganglion cells, but these populations decrease with proliferation and maturation of the chromaffin cell population during the first years of life in the human. The pheochromocytes are arranged in nests and cords and contain abundant membrane-bound dense granules, in which the catecholamines are stored. On stimulation, these granules are transported to the cell surface via the microtubular system, and the neurotransmitter contents of the vesicles released by exocytosis. Although circulating epinephrine is derived entirely from the adrenal medulla, only about 30% of the circulating norepinephrine comes from the medulla. The rest is released from nerve terminals and hence the adrenal medulla is not essential for life.

1.2 Functions of medullary catecholamines

The physiologic effects of epinephrine and norepinephrine are initiated by their binding to adrenergic receptors on the surface of target cells. These receptors are prototypical examples of seven-pass transmembrane proteins that are coupled to G proteins which stimulate or inhibit intracellular signaling pathways. Complex physiologic responses result from adrenal medullary stimulation because there are multiple receptor types which are differentially expressed in different tissues and cells. The alpha and beta adrenergic receptors and their subtypes were originally defined by differential binding of various agonists/antagonists and by analysis of molecular clones.

In general, circulating epinephrine and norepinephrine released from the adrenal medulla have the same effects on target organs as direct stimulation by sympathetic nerves, except the effects last five to ten times as long because these neurotransmitter hormones are removed too slowly from peripheral circulation. Additionally, of course, circulating hormones can cause effects in cells and tissues that are not directly innervated. The physiologic consequences of medullary catecholamine release are justifiably framed as responses which aid in dealing with stress. These effects are important in helping the body to react to emergency situations, thus norepinephrine and epinephrine are sometimes called the hormones of "fight or flight". A listing of some major effects mediated by medullary catecholamine are: increased rate and force of contraction of the heart muscle; constriction of blood vessels (this causes widespread vasoconstriction, resulting in increased resistance and hence arterial blood pressure); dilation of bronchioles (assists in pulmonary ventilation); stimulation of lipolysis in fat cells (this provides fatty acids for energy production in many tissues and aids in conservation of dwindling reserves of blood glucose); increased metabolic rate (oxygen consumption and heat production increase throughout the body as well as the breakdown of glycogen in skeletal muscle which provides glucose for energy production); dilation of the pupils; inhibition of certain "non-essential" processes: an example is inhibition of gastrointestinal secretion and motor activity. Common stimuli for secretion of adrenomedullary hormones include exercise, hypoglycemia, hemorrhage and emotional distress.

1.3 Tumours of the adrenal medulla: pheochromocytomas

A tumour cell is part of a tissue that is abnormally growing. It may be either malignant or benign in nature. "Tumour" originally meant "swelling" because, with unchecked cellular reproduction, the tissue affected swells to sometimes grotesque proportions. Tumour cells that are malignant are generally referred to as cancer cells, and have the ability to metastasize, or spread to neighboring tissues and grow tumours there. Benign tumour cells do not invade neighboring tissues, but may grow to great size and cause other problems: breathing, mobility, circulatory. While a malignant tumour might not be eradicated by surgically removing it, a benign tumour generally is.

Tumours of the adrenal gland can develop in either the cortex or the medulla. Benign tumours of the cortex are called adrenal cortical adenomas. Malignant tumours are called adrenal cortical carcinomas. The World Health Organization reserves the term pheochromocytoma for tumours arising from chromaffin cells in the adrenal medulla. A small number of phaeochromocytomas start outside the medulla part of the adrenal gland and are known as extra-adrenal phaeochromocytomas or paragangliomas. A pheochromocytoma is an intra-adrenal sympathetic paraganglioma. This arbitrary nomenclature emphasizes important distinctive properties of intra-adrenal tumours, including an often adrenergic phenotype, relatively low rate of malignancy, and predilection to occur in particular hereditary syndromes. Although pheochromocytomas are extremely rare in humans, with an annual incidence of less than 1 per million, occult germline mutations characteristic of familial syndromes are now found in more than 20% of patients with apparently sporadic tumours, bringing the percentage of tumours with a known genetic basis close to 30% (Karagiannis et al., 2007). In addition, tumour location and risk of malignancy vary with the underlying genetic defect.

Pheochromocytoma develops as a single tumour or as more than one growth. Only one adrenal gland is usually affected. Rarely, tumours affect both adrenal glands; these are known as bilateral adrenal tumours. The tumours may occur at any age, but they are most common from early to mid-adulthood. In patients with pheochromocytomas, there is a release of excessive amounts of catecholamines. If the diagnosis of a pheochromocytoma is overlooked, the consequences could be disastrous, even fatal; however, if a pheochromocytoma is found, it is potentially curable. Most pheochromocytomas are benign (noncancerous), and 90% of cases can be successfully treated by surgery (Petri et al., 2009).

Many cardiac manifestations are associated with pheochromocytomas. Hypertension is the most common complication. Cardiac arrhythmias, such as atrial and ventricular fibrillation, may occur because of excessive plasma catecholamine levels. Other complications include myocarditis, signs and symptoms of myocardial infarction, dilated cardiomyopathy, and pulmonary edema, either of cardiac or noncardiac origin. Different neurologic complications may also occur. A pheochromocytoma-induced hypertensive crisis may precipitate hypertensive encephalopathy, which is characterized by altered mental status, focal neurologic signs and symptoms, or seizures. Other neurologic complications include stroke due to cerebral infarction or an embolic event secondary to a mural thrombus from a dilated cardiomyopathy. Moreover, intracerebral hemorrhage may origine because of uncontrolled hypertension.

2. Pheochromocytoma cell lines

Pheochromocytoma cells rapidly cease proliferating in primary culture. In most instances, proliferation of neoplastic chromaffin cells ceases with two weeks and does not resume, although the cells persist in cultures maintained for many months (Tischler et al., 2004). In addition, variable proportions of the tumour cell populations undergo spontaneous neuronal differentiation. Propensity for neuronal differentiation may in part reflect underlying genetic abnormalities. Establishment of pheochromocytoma cell lines is therefore a challenging task. Routinely, different immunocytochemical staining provide a means for distinguishing neoplastic chromaffin cells from other cell types in primary cultures and for rapidly assessing the success of attempts to establish cell lines (Powers et al., 2000).

The development of experimental applications of animal models of pheochromocytoma has, to a large extent, been initially driven by intriguing observations made with human tumour tissue. Individual animal models have subsequently found their own applications, while at the same time contributing, in different ways and varying degrees, to understanding of human pathology. The rarity of pheochromocytomas is notable across species, with the exception of the rat. In some strains of laboratory rats, upwards of 30% of males spontaneously develop pheochromocytomas. In contrast, the lifetime frequency of the tumours is typically around 1% in wildtype laboratory mice, but much higher in several genetically engineered mouse models (Ohta et al., 2006; Tischler et al., 2004). Similarities and differences between the rat and mouse models suggest both parallel and unique applications for each and also raise questions of which model is more relevant to various aspects of human tumour biology. Advantages of the murine models include genetic resemblances to human pheochromocytomas (Eaton & Duplan, 2004; Molatore et al., 2010). Disadvantages include an apparently less stable phenotype.

At present, a variety of continuous adrenal medullary cell lines have been established (Eaton & Duplan, 2004). Initially, continuous chromaffin cell lines were derived from spontaneous pheochromocytoma tumours of the medulla, either from murine (i.e., rat PC12 cells) or human sources. In particular, the first continuous cell line derived from a sporadic benign human adrenal pheochomocytoma is the KNA cell line (Pfragner et al., 1998) although earlier attempts by these same researchers resulted in four similar human cell lines with finite lifespans of up to one year in culture. However, there is a heterogeneity among KNA subclones. In addition, KNA cells detach early from the tissue culture dish and grow as large multicellular spheroids with loose cell-cell adhesion. A similar medullary adrenal cell line derived from a human pheochromocytoma is the KAT45 cell line (Venihaki et al., 1998). Such cell lines have revealed both the unique characteristics of oncogenic adrenal medullary tumours, as well as similarities in catecholamine regulation to normal chromaffin adrenal tissue. However, both human cell lines have only provided *in vitro* data and it is generally accepted that there are currently no adequately documented human pheochromocytoma cell lines, despite the attempts to establish them.

Over the last few decades, more sophisticated molecular methods have allowed for induced tumourigenesis and targeted oncogenesis *in vivo*, where isolation of specific populations of mouse cell lines of endocrine origin have resulted in model cells to examine a variety of regulatory pathways in the chromaffin phenotype (Eaton & Duplan, 2004; Tischler et al., 2004). Although these cells are attractive experimental models by virtue of their genetic and functional similarities to human pheochromocytomas, a drawback compared to other models is a greater tendency to phenotype drift. This may in part be due to the same factors that cause mouse pheochromocytomas to appear polymorphous in histologic sections or it may reflect cell culture artefact. Finally, conditional immortalization with retroviral infection of chromaffin precursors has provided homogeneous and expandable chromaffin cells in animal models. This same strategy of immortalization with conditionally expressed oncogenes has been expanded to create the first disimmortalizable chromaffin cells (Eaton & Duplan, 2004). However, these promising lines have not been extensively studied, yet.

Although the available cell models have already been used for several additional novel applications, they are best regarded as complementary systems of human pheochromocytomas. Data indicates that caution is warranted in drawing general conclusions from any single cell line, but also suggest that understanding of factors that permit pheochromocytoma cells to proliferate might itself provide important insights for tumour biology.

2.1 PC12 cells

Among chromaffin cell lines, the earliest example is PC12 rat cell line. It was first established from a representative rat pheochromocytoma in 1976 (Greene & Tischler, 1976) and has become an important workhorse in many disciplines. PC12 cells arose from animals that had been irradiated postnatally, probably with resultant genetic damage that permitted the lines to be established. The phenotype of the PC12 line has been remarkably stable during almost 35 years of propagation. However, a somewhat variability of different desired traits has occurred in some laboratories, emphasizing the importance of freezing and storing early passages of any cell line. The characteristics of the cells have also been affected by culture conditions, most notably a switch made in some laboratories early in the history of the cell line from RPMI 1640 medium to Dulbecco's modified Eagle's medium, which increases cell flattening and cell-substratum adhesion.

The popularity of PC12 cells is mainly because of their extreme versatility for pharmacological manipulation, their ease of culture and the large amount of background knowledge on their proliferation and differentiation. Like adrenal chromaffin cells, PC12 cells synthesize and store dopamine and sometimes noradrenaline, which are released upon depolarization in a Ca^{2+}-dependent way. A common application of PC12 cells concerns the study of the cellular and molecular aspects of cell death, involving normal and neoplastic conditions. Also, a notable characteristic of PC12 cells is that they can readily be induced to differentiate in culture with the NGF, whereby cells cease to multiply, assume a neurite-bearing phenotype that resemble mature sympathetic neurons and exhibit firm attachment to the substratum.

3. Apoptosis in pheochromocytoma PC12 cells

The fate of a cell is determined by a balance of survival or promoting signals. While survival signals mediate cell maintenance, promoting signals induce cells to proliferate, differentiate, transform or apoptose. The natural occurrence of cell death has long been appreciated and was widely studied by nineteenth century biologists. While multiple modes of cell death have been described, undoubtedly the most renowned process is the programmed form of cell death known as apoptosis. In many diseases, aberrant regulation of apoptosis is the central abnormality. For example, resistance of cells to apoptosis is thought to be responsible for many types of cancer, while on the other hand in many neurological disorders an excessive neuronal death is a central feature.

As NGF can readily induce PC12 transition from a naïve, actively proliferating to a quiescent, differentiated phenotype, the responsiveness to NGF by PC12 cells has allowed them to be used for a great variety of studies concerning not only PC12 cells as a purported model of adrenal medullary cells, but as a model of neuronal differentiation and pluripotency. These features are possessed by primitive progenitors from the medulla which can differentiate into either chromaffin cells or sympathetic neurons, depending on the local microenvironment.

A search of the PubMed database in June 2011 yields almost 1800 papers published from 1990 describing apoptosis in PC12 cells. Indeed, PC12 is considered a suitable and reliable model to study (neuro)apoptotic mechanisms as well as for predicting (neuro)cytotoxicity of experimental drugs and natural compounds. Although caution is warranted in drawing general conclusions from any single cell line, understanding of factors that modulate PC12 cell proliferation/death might itself provide important insights in cell biology.

In this section, we will concentrate on the programmed cell death mechanisms in PC12 cells, considering primarily the recent insights achieved in the last years. We will also consider these mechanisms under a pharmacological point of view, as for instance in the context of (neuro)cytotoxicological studies and/or the developing of promising compounds with potential therapeutic applications.

3.1 Cellular machinery

Apoptosis, also known as programmed cell death, is characterized by distinctive stereotyped morphological and biochemical alterations, such as exposure of phosphatidylserine on the outer leaflet of the plasma membrane and blebbing, cell shrinkage, chromatin condensation, and DNA fragmentation. This process leads to the formation of apoptotic bodies that are subsequently eliminated by phagocytosis. Key event in the apoptotic process is the activation of caspases, a family of cysteinyl aspartate-specific proteases. They are constitutively expressed in almost all cell types as inactive proenzymes (zymogens) that became processed and activated in response to a variety of pro-apoptotic stimuli. Evidence for the sequential activation of caspases has lead to the concept of a caspase cascade: during apoptosis, apoptogenic stimuli induce the autocatalitically activation of initiator caspases; subsequentely they cleave and thereby activate downstream effector caspases that carry on the cleavage of specific proteins in order to "dismantle" the cell.

The induction of apoptosis can be mediated by two pathways: the death receptor-dependent or the mitochondria-dependent pathways, also known as the extrinsic and intrinsic apoptotic pathways, respectively (Jin & El-Deiry, 2005). The extrinsic apoptotic pathway begins at the cell surface where death receptors bind their ligands, such TNF family members, including FasL (or CD95L). Ligand binding to the death receptor triggers the oligomerization of the death receptor and the aggregation of the characteristic intracellular motif, known as "death domain" able to recruit adaptor proteins containing death domains, such as FADD. These adaptor proteins function to activate initiator caspase-8 and/or caspase-10, resulting in the formation of the death-inducing signaling complex. Activated initiator caspases in turn process and activate the downstream executioner caspases, including caspase-3, -6, and -7, which execute the destruction of the cell (Degterev et al., 2003). The study of death receptors-induced apoptosis in PC12 cells has been particularly important in understanding the pathogenesis of neurodegenerative diseases. For instance, it is of interest to note that amyloid β peptide toxicity (a model of Alzheimer disease *in vitro*, see also below) may involve the CD95 pathway while TNF is strictly linked with excitotoxic mechanisms. The intrinsic apoptotic pathway involves the mitochondria in response to diverse cellular stress such as UV and gamma irradiation, heat and the activation of some oncogenic factors. The critical event in the mitochondria-mediated apoptotic pathway is the mitochondrial outer membrane permeabilization, that prompts the release of various proteins of the mitochondrial intermembrane space into the cytosol. In addition, the mitochondrial proteins of Bcl2 family (i.e., Bcl2 and Bax) play a fundamental role as negative or positive modulators. Of importance, cytochrome c, released from mitochondria, binds to Apaf-1 to form a complex, the "apoptosome," that recruits procaspase-9 and facilitates its oligomerization and activation. Activated caspase-9, in turn, processes and activates the executioner caspases-3, -6, and -7, which drive the execution of the cell.

The homeostasis of healthy tissues is maintained by the survival signaling pathways responsible for the control of cell proliferation. In this respect, one of the best-studied mechanism responsible for apoptosis in PC12-derived neurons is the serum or growth factor withdrawal leading to the classical apoptosis. In contrast, the best-characterized survival pathway in PC12 cells is that involving NGF. NGF belongs to a family of structurally related neurotrophin proteins, including BDNF, NT-3, and NT-4/5 that function to support the growth and survival of many populations of neurons. NGF binds the TrkA neurotrophin receptor, whereas BDNF and NT-4/5 bind the TrkB neurotrophin receptor, and NT-3 primarily binds the TrkC neurotrophin receptor. These Trk neurotrophin receptors are able to protect neuronal cells from apoptosis, and they can stimulate neuronal regeneration in different model systems._NGF activates a variety of signaling cascades, including the protein kinases ERK1/2 and PI3K-Akt pathways, that are dynamically linked to the apoptotic machinery in a complex cellular signaling network. Their activation by survival signals serves to block apoptotic signaling. The proto-oncogene protein kinase Raf-MEK-ERK1/2 pathway is the better characterized Ras (a GTPase) effector pathway that plays a key role in PC12 cell proliferation. Once activated, ERK phosphorylates and thereby regulates the activities of a number of substrates, including multiple transcription factors inducing alteration in gene expression directly linked with the extracellular signal from the cell surface receptors and thus preventing apoptosis. It is very recent the discovery that, among all the targets of NGF-activated ERK in PC12 cells the two microRNA 221 and 222 are involved in NGF-dependent neuronal survival. (Terasawa et al., 2009). In PC12 cells, the PI3K-Akt pathway, the other downstream mediator of NGF, includes, among its several targets, the FoxO family of transcription factors which play a particularly important role in the regulation of cell death, proliferation, and survival through modulation of the expression of cell-cycle inhibitory genes and pro-apoptotic genes. The kinase Akt also controls the activity of mTORC1, another key mediator of cell growth, proliferation, and survival that can function to inhibit PC12 cell apoptosis.

Another intriguing issue, recently demonstrated in several models including PC12, is that cell cycle activation often precedes neuronal death , indicating that neurons attempt to divide before dying (Bianco et al., 2011). Multiple pathways and stimuli, including NGF deprivation, have been demonstrated to participate in the regulation of cell cycle events during death of differentiated PC12. These aspects may have a significant clinical interest. Indeed, different papers have reported the re-expression of proteins of the cell cycle in neurons from patients with Alzheimer disease, Parkinson's disease, ataxia telangiectasia, stroke, and other neurodegenerative conditions.

On the other hand, controversial is the use of PC12 as model of apoptotis induced by the release of the excitatory neurotransmitter glutamate. For many years PC12 cells have been used to investigate NMDA receptor mediated excitotoxicity and potential neuroprotective mechanisms (Lee et al., 2006). In a key paper, Casado and coll. (Casado et al., 1996) demonstrated an increase in NR1 protein (a NMDA channel subunit) expression levels in PC12 cells in response to NGF, and their ability to evoke NMDA and glutamate induced currents. However, other studies are not entirely consistent with these results. Among them, Edwards and coll. (Edwards et al., 2007) demonstrated the absence of functional NMDA receptors in PC12 cells thus suggesting that the mechanism by which NMDA or glutamate induces excitotoxicity in PC12 cells cannot be assumed to occurr by direct actions on NMDA receptors but, instead, non-NMDA receptor mechanisms, including oxidative stress, may drive cytotoxic response to high glutamate concentrations.

PC12 cells have been also shown to be useful models to characterize the molecular mechanisms that determine cellular commitment to cell death following oxygen-derived

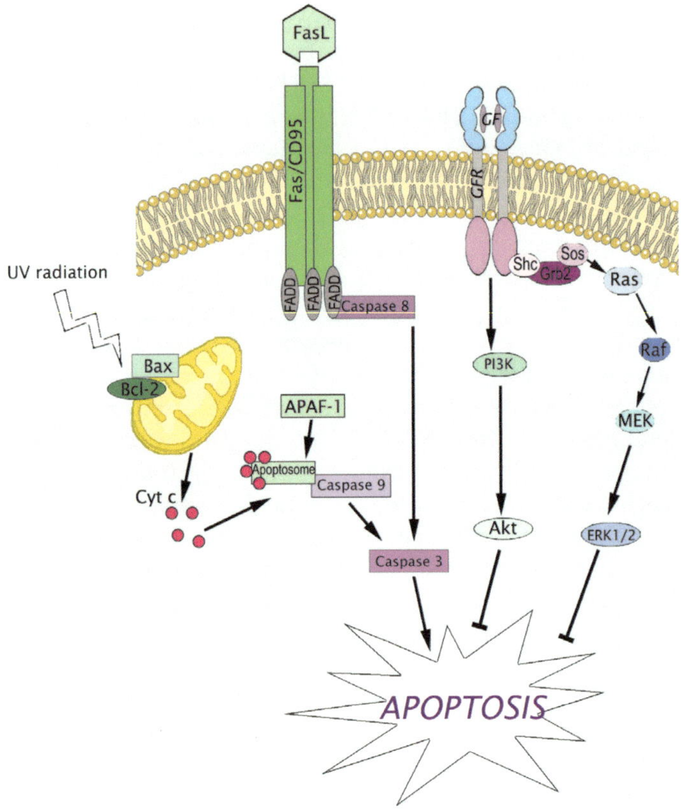

Fig. 1. Scheme of some apoptotic mechanisms achieved in PC12 cells (GF: Growth factors; GFR: GF receptors; Shc/Grb2/Sos: classical protein complex involved in Ras activation).

free radicals including superoxide, peroxynitrite, peroxyl radicals, and the hydroxyl radical. The toxicity of oxygen-derived free radicals arises from the presence of one or more unpaired electrons that extract electrons from macromolecules, ultimately inactivating them. At high level reactive oxygene species induce the oxidation of protein, lipid and DNA/RNA, increase the leakage of lactate dehydrogenase and reduce the intracellular glutathione level. In neuron and in neuronal cell lines (e.g., PC12) accumulation of H_2O_2 can activate the stress sensor JNK/p38 MAPK pathway (Cho et al., 2008) and eventually the tumour suppressor gene p53 (Reuter et al., 2010). A source of the hydroxyl radical is also the nitrogen-derived radical, nitric oxide, which can combine with superoxide to produce peroxynitrite. Peroxynitrite is capable of directly damaging proteins, lipids, and nucleic acids and can generate hydroxyl radicals and NO_2 in PC12 cells (Pytlowany et al., 2008; Shacka et al., 2006).

In the last decade increasing attention has been focused on alternative signaling pathways leading to cell death, as for instance autophagy and parthanatos. In PC12 cells serum or growth factors withdrawal can lead to autophagy instead of apoptosis. Autophagy is an evolutionarily conserved lysosomal pathway involved in the turnover of long-lived proteins and organelles. Functions of autophagy include: remodeling during development and differentiation and elimination of unwanted or damaged organelles and molecules. These functions are important for maintenance of cytoplasmic homeostasis. Autophagy can be stimulated in response to different situations of stress, such as starvation, changes in cell volume, oxidative stress, accumulation of misfolded proteins, hormonal signaling, irradiation, xenobiotic or the pro-apoptotic ligand TRAIL treatment. Following the induction of autophagy, autophagic vesicles or autophagosomes are formed through the assembly and expansion of double-layered, membrane-bound structures of endoplasmic reticulum around whole organelles and isolated proteins. The autophagosome encapsulates the cytosolic materials, then docks and fuses with lysosomes or other vacuoles, causing degradation of the autophagosomal contents. At the molecular level, the signaling pathway that leads to autophagy seem to involve the activities of PI3K and mTOR. In PC12 cells, two key autophagy genes, ATG7 and beclin 1, have been recently reported to be involved in this non-apoptotic death pathway.

In traumatic brain injury, excitotoxicity, ischemia, and, in many neurodegenerative disorders, PARP-1 activation is an early biochemical cell death event. PARP-1 activation leads to a unique form of cell death that is in large part mediated via accumulation of PAR and nuclear translocation of AIF from mitochondria that induces large-scale DNA fragmentation, chromatin condensation, and cell death. PARP-1-dependent cell death is caspase independent as caspase inhibitors are ineffective in limiting it and is termed parthanatos. In several neuronal model including PC12, parthanatos has been recently studied together with its players (Kondo et al., 2010). The intriguing aspect emerging from parthanatos is that the nuclear–mitochondrial cross talk with PAR is important player for cell death initiation. Indeed, PAR is generated mainly in the nucleus and localizes to cytosol and interacts with mitochondria to induce cell death. Parthanatos is a unique form of cell death that occurs across organ systems, which is primarily mediated by toxic accumulation of PAR in cytosol from overactivation of PARP-1. Although the mechanism of parthanatos includes PAR as a signaling molecule to induce AIF release from mitochondria, the mechanistic aspects of the AIF-releasing capacity of PAR remain unclear.

Although programmed cell death is well accepted as a common homeostatic property of all tissues, its frequency is underestimated. Dying cells are rarely observed in normal tissues, thus illustrating the effectiveness of the clearance process. Indeed, a key event in the apoptosis programme is the swift clearance and phagocytosis of dying cells by wandering or resident scavengers and neighbouring phagocytes (Gregory & Pound, 2011). However, the vast majority of research on apoptosis has focused on the stages leading up to the clearance phase, or indeed has been carried out under artificial conditions lacking the clearance phase such as in model populations of non-phagocytic cells *in vitro*. In normal or pathological tissues, apoptotic cells are invariably found in association with macrophages and neighbouring cells of various lineages which actively engage in the apoptotic cell clearance process. In the developing brain, multipotential cells phagocytose their dying neighbours prior to the appearance of the specialist phagocytes of the nervous system, the microglia. Furthermore, in tumours, clearance of apoptotic cells is mediated by macrophages, non-macrophage stromal cells, and tumour cells themselves. These features need to be taken into account in elucidating the finer mechanisms of apoptotic cell death, as for instance those underlying the interactions of the apoptotic cell with its environment.

3.2 Factors and compounds involved in apoptosis regulation

Much current work with *in vitro* systems for (neuro)cytotoxicity/(neuro)cytoprotection testing lies in maximizing their potential for yelding valid mechanistic response. Among the advantages of *in vitro* models, i.e., PC12 cells, are the option to study a single cell type of interest in the absence of other cell types, ease of direct observation and measurement of cellular responses to chemicals, a defined extracellular environment, and direct interactions of the chemical with test cells. Until recently, it was thought that cytotoxic/cytoprotective drugs affected target cells directly by interfering with some life-maintaining function. However, of late, it has been shown that exposure to several drugs with disparate mechanisms of action modulates apoptosis in both pathological and normal cells.

Among ubiquitous toxic environmental contaminants, cadmium, manganese, copper (an essential trace element contained in common foods), methylmercury, and bisphenol A may induce apoptosis in PC12 cells. Recently, it has been demonstrated that melamine, which has been used in milk powder as an additive to raise the measured protein content, and monocrotophos, a widely used organophosphate pesticide, also displayed apoptotic effects. In contrast, the phenol tert-butylhydroquinone, a synthetic food grade antioxidant, that is used to stabilize foods, fats and vegetable oils aganist oxidative damage, prevents apoptosis in differentiated PC12 cells. Similar effects are achieved by pyrroloquinoline quinone, a novel redox cofactor which exists in various foods.

Current evidence in the literature supports a cytoprotective role of NGF in PC12 cells (see also above) such as against apoptosis induced by TNFα. The transition of cells from a proliferative to a differentiated, quiescent stage is associated with acquisition of a highly reduced intracellular environment, which confers cytoprotection against oxidative challenge. The reason as to why PC12 cells acquire a reduced intracellular status during differentiation is probably due to the fact that neuronal cells are highly oxidative, which could render cells vulnerable to reactive oxygene species-induced injury. Therefore, adaptation of differentiated neuron-like PC12 cells to a reduced environment and a higher expression of redox enzymes would permit cells to function optimally under oxidizing conditions, and increase the likelihood for survival against oxidative challenges.

Oxidative stress has been widely believed to be an important pathogenetic mechanism of neuronal apoptosis, occurring in different brain diseases, as for instance Alzheimer disease and Parkinson's disease. It is thus not surprising that neuron-like PC12 cells are extensively used in the study of brain disorders. In this respect, amyloid β peptide, dopamine, 6-hydroxydopamine, and MPP^+ are shown to induce apoptosis in PC12 cells. Amyloid β peptide toxicity is a well-established pathway of neuronal cell death which play a role in Alzheimer's disease. In addition, 6-hydroxydopamine is a neurotoxin used by scientists to selectively kill dopaminergic and noradrenergic neurons. The main use for 6-hydroxydopamine in scientific research is to induce Parkinsonism, as well as the neurotoxin 1-methyl-4-phenylpyridinium. Similarly, dieldrin, which may selectively destroy dopaminergic neurons, induces apoptosis in PC12 cells. It is a chlorinated hydrocarbon originally produced as an insecticide and has been reported to be one of the environmental factors correlated with Parkinson's disease. The effects of some of these substances can be reverted by different anti-apoptotic compounds. Among them, some novel substituted bisphenol A derivatives, bone morphogenetic protein 7, and galantamine have protective effects against amyloid β peptide-induced PC12 apoptosis. Galantamine is an acetylcholinesterase inhibitor widely used for patients with Alzheimer's disease. In addition, granulocyte-macrophage colony-stimulating factor, a hematopoietic cytokine that has the potential for clinical application, significantly reduces 1-methyl-4-phenylpyridinium-induced PC12 apoptosis. Some interesting results may also account from gene therapy strategies. For instance, the anti-apoptotic herpes simplex virus type 2 gene

ICP10PK has been reported to protect neuronally differentiated PC12 cells from apoptosis death caused by MPP+. Finally, other substances which display somewhat activity in brain have been shown to modulate apoptosis in PC12 cells: the opioid morphine induces apoptosis, while lithium chloride, the antipsychotics citalopram and trifluoperazine, and serotonin exert opposite effects.

name	description	source	effect
hydroxyecdysone	ecdysteroid hormone	different plant sources	anti-apoptotic
apocynum leaf	flavonoid extract	*Apocynum venetum*	anti-apoptotic
aucubin	iridoid glycoside	*Aucuba japonica* and other plant sources	anti-apoptotic
camptothecin	alkaloid	*Camptotheca accuminata*	apoptotic
cEppt		cinnamon extract	anti-apoptotic
decursin	coumarin	*Angelica gigas*	anti-apoptotic
euplotin C	sesquiterpenoid	ciliate protist *Euplotes crassus*	apoptotic
gomesin	peptide	tarantula *Acanthoscurria gomesiana*	apoptotic
ginsenoside Rb1	steroid glycoside	ginseng (*Panax*)	anti-apoptotic
icariin	flavonoid	*Epimedium brevicornum*	anti-apoptotic
isochaihulactone	lignan compound	*Bupleurum scorzonerifolium*	anti-apoptotic
isoflavones	poliphenolic compounds	*Fabaceae*	anti-apoptotic
kaempferol	flavonoid	different plant sources	anti-apoptotic
lactacystin	cyclic amide	bacteria *Streptomyces*	apoptotic
MAM	naphthoquinone	*Polygonum cuspidatum*	anti-apoptotic
olive leaf		olive tree (*Olea europaea*)	anti-apoptotic
paclitaxel/docetaxel	taxanes	*Taxus brevifolia, baccata*	apoptotic
paeoniflorin	monoterpene glycoside	*Paeonia albiflora*	anti-apoptotic
puerarin	isoflavone C-glycoside	*Pueraria lobota*	anti-apoptotic
quercetin	flavonoid	*Quercum* and other plant sources	anti-apoptotic
salidroside	phenylpropanoid glycoside	*Rhodiola rosea*	anti-apoptotic
schisandrin B/C	lignans	*Schisandra chinensis*	anti-apoptotic
SG-168	acetal skeleton	*Dendrobium nobile*	anti-apoptotic
silibinin	flavonolignan	milk thistle (*Silybum arianum*)	anti-apoptotic
tetrahydroxystilbene glucoside	monomer of stilbene	*Polygonum multiflorum*	anti-apoptotic
trans resveratrol	phenol	grapes	anti-apoptotic
vincristine/vinblastine	vinca alkaloids	*Catharanthus roseus*	apoptotic
xyloketals		mangrove fungus *Xylaria*	anti-apoptotic

Table 1. Examples of natural products identified as modulators of PC12 cell apoptosis

Many commercialized drugs have been obtained by the synthesis of new compounds. On the other hand, an alternative source of drugs is natural products (and the structural modification of natural products), which frequently seem to be more effective and/or less toxic. A natural product is a chemical compound or substance produced by a living organism - found in nature that usually has a pharmacological or biological activity. Nature is an attractive source of new therapeutic candidate compounds (da Rocha et al., 2001) as a tremendous chemical diversity is found in millions of species of plants, animals, marine organisms and microorganisms. For many living organisms, this chemical diversity reflects the impact of evolution in the selection and conservation of self-defense mechanisms that represent the strategies employed to repel or destroy predators. However, the development of novel agents from natural sources presents obstacles that are not usually met when one deals with synthetic compounds. For instance, there may be difficulties in accessing the source of the samples, obtaining appropriate amounts of the sample, identification and isolation of the active compound in the sample, and problems in synthesizing the necessary amounts of the compound of interest. These problems became evident when the tubulin-interacting agent taxol was introduced in clinical use. Antitumour activity was observed in various *in vitro* systems, including PC12 cells, and *in vivo* tumours. It took some years to develop a semi-synthetic analog which is derived from a renewable source. Currently, total synthesis has been achieved drug supply is no longer a problem. Among their various biological activities, natural products can modulate apoptosis signaling pathways (Fulda, 2010). In PC12 cells, many scientific papers report pro-apoptotic and anti-apoptotic activity of different natural products, isolated mostly from plant sources, others from microbes, fungi and different marine organisms. Table 1 shows some examples of agents derived from natural sources which have been studied in 2010-2011 as modulators of PC12 cell apoptosis. Some "classical" apoptotic modulators have been also indicated.

In many studies, PC12 cell models to study apoptotic mechanisms/modulations have been obtained with the use of lipopolysaccharide, the major component of the outer membrane of Gram-negative bacteria, or ethanol. Apoptosis can be also induced by depletion of serum and NGF from the culture medium. Other factors may include glucose deprivation, a high oxygen atmosphere or oxidative agents as for instance hydrogen peroxide, peroxynitrite, the lipid peroxidation product 4-hydroxynonenal, and 7-ketocholesterol, the major oxidation product of cholesterol found in human atherosclerotic plaque. Moreover, many other organic/endogenous compounds, like parathyroid hormone(1-34), corticosterone, and ceramide exert pro-apoptotic effects in PC12 cells. Interestingly, taurine, a free amino acid with antioxidant activity present in high concentrations in a variety of organs of mammalians, protects cells from apoptosis induced by hydrogen peroxide. In addition, heparin-binding epidermal growth factor-like growth factor is a member of the epidermal growth factor family that is expressed in many cell types. In PC12 cells, its protective effects against apoptosis induced by oxygen and glucose deprivation has been reported. Recently, different synthetic compounds have been shown to display cytoprotective behaviours against oxidative stress, among them folacin C60, the isothiocyanates 3H-1, 2-dithiole-3-thione, fasudil mesylate, the new 1,2,4-triazine, , 3-butyl-6-bromo-1(3H)-isobenzofuranon and a new synthetic 1,2-diaryl oxazine derivative, 2-ethoxy-4,5-diphenyl-1,3-oxazine-6-one. In this line, the soluble guanylyl cyclase activator YC-1, which inhibits the hypoxia-inducible factor 1, and edaravone, a potent free radical scavenger in clinical use, significantly antagonize the PC12 apoptosis induced by glutamate or prion protein peptides, respectively.

The ability to induce apoptosis in many tumoural systems, including PC12 cells, has been reported as key property for different chemotherapeutic drugs or substances with potential therapeutic activity. For instance, the chemotherapeutic drugs fluorouracil, paclitaxel, and enediynes are potent inducers of apoptosis in PC12 cells. Also, therapeutic concentrations of cisplatin may cause a hybrid type of cell death characterized by concurrent apoptosis and necrosis in the same individual cells. Interestingly, I-387, a novel synthetic compound that inhibits tubulin action and exhibits potent antitumour activity in various preclinical models, has been shown to display apoptotic activity in different systems, including PC12 cells, suggesting that it may represent a new antimitotic agent for management of various malignancies. It is also of interest the fact that human pheochromocytomas express high levels of the receptor subtype 2 for the neuropeptide somatostatin. Recently, it has been demonstrated that somatostatin agonists as well as somatostatin cytotoxic compounds may induce PC12 cell apoptosis, although no data are available on pheochromocytomas *in vivo* (Ziegler et al., 2009). Generally, the implications of such apoptotic studies in oncology are puzzling. Indeed, often forgotten in the biology of tumours, cell loss in malignant disease is a very significant component of tumour dynamics. One may assume that enhanced apoptosis will retard tumour growth and hence indicate a favourable prognosis compared with tumours showing a low apoptotic activity. However, also the opposite seems to be true: apoptosis is a common process in high-grade malignancy, with high apoptosis indices generally reflecting poor prognosis. Clearly, the balance between cell birth and cell death must favour the former in order for a tumour to grow but, given the properties of apoptotic cells and their capacity to affect their microenvironments and host immune systems, it seems likely that the cell-death programme also provides oncogenic drive (Gregory & Pound, 2011). In this respect, the implications that the homeostatic properties of apoptosis can be hijacked as a sinister, facilitatory mechanism for malignant disease development and progression are clear and the programme may be regarded as 'altruistic' in this context: loss of a fraction of the growing population for the greater good of the whole (but detriment of the host).

4. Conclusion

From a general point of view, dysregulation of apoptosis is associated with many pathologic conditions and may even be central in the pathogenesis of many diseases (Zangemeister-Wittke & Simon, 2001). Apoptosis research is rapidly proceeding making it difficult to keep track of the constant stream of newly identified proteins and molecular interactions involved in cell death regulation. However, there is a general agreement that the suppression, overexpression or mutation of a number of factors which orchestrate the apoptotic process are associated with disease. As outlined above, the study of apoptosis mechanisms in PC12 cells represent one application currently of great potential interest.

In pheochromocytomas as well as in the majority of malignancy there is a need of novel compounds which may act as potent and selective apoptotic modulators. In the clinical practice of benign pheochromocytoma, the most common treatment is surgical removal of the entire affected adrenal gland. On the other hand, there is currently no effective treatment for malignant pheochromocytoma. Radiotherapy provides benefit in some patients with malignant pheochromocytoma. Chemotherapy with cyclophosphamide, vincristine, and dacarbazine may produce partial remission, but again is not curative. In this respect, much work is still to do in order to exploit new chemical space for drug-like molecules.

5. Abbreviations

AIF, apoptosis inducing factor; *Apaf-1*, apoptosis protease-activating factor 1; *BDNF*, brain-derived neurotrophic factor; *ERK*, extracellular-regulated kinases; *FADD*, Fas-associated death domain; *FasL*, Fas Ligand; *FoxO*, forkhead box O; *GTP*, guanosine triphosphate; *JNK*, Jun N-terminal Kinase; *MAPK*, mitogen-activated protein kinases; *MEK*, MAPK kinases; *MPP*$^+$, 1-methyl-4-phenylpyridinium; *mTOR*, mammalian target of rapamycin; *mTORC1*, mTOR complex 1; *NGF*, Nerve Growth Factor; *NMDA*, N-Methyl-D-aspartic acid; *NT*, neurotrophin; *PARP-1*, poly (ADP-ribose) polymerase-1; *PI3K*, phosphatidylinositol 3-kinases; *TNF*, Tumour Necrosis Factor; *Trk*, transmembrane tyrosine kinase proteins.

6. References

Bianco, M.R., Berbenni, M., Amara, F., Viggiani, S., Fragni, M., Galimberti, V., Colombo, D., Cirillo, G., Papa, M., Alberghina, L., & Colangelo, A.M. (2011). Cross-talk between cell cycle induction and mitochondrial dysfunction during oxidative stress and nerve growth factor withdrawal in differentiated PC12 cells. *J Neurosci Res*, Vol.89, No.8, pp. 1302-1315

Casado, M., Lopez-Guajardo, A., Mellstrom, B., Naranjo, J.R., & Lerma, J. (1996). Functional N-methyl-D-aspartate receptors in clonal rat phaeochromocytoma cells. *J Physiol*, Vol.490 (Pt 2), pp. 391-404

Cho, E.S., Lee, K.W., & Lee, H.J. (2008). Cocoa procyanidins protect PC12 cells from hydrogen-peroxide-induced apoptosis by inhibiting activation of p38 MAPK and JNK. *Mutat Res*, Vol.640, No.1-2, pp. 123-130

da Rocha, A.B., Lopes, R.M., & Schwartsmann, G. (2001). Natural products in anticancer therapy. *Curr Opin Pharmacol*, Vol.1, No.4, pp. 364-369

Degterev, A., Boyce, M., & Yuan, J. (2003). A decade of caspases. *Oncogene*, Vol.22, No.53, pp. 8543-8567

Eaton, M.J., & Duplan, H. (2004). Useful cell lines derived from the adrenal medulla. *Mol Cell Endocrinol*, Vol.228, No.1-2, pp. 39-52

Edwards, M.A., Loxley, R.A., Williams, A.J., Connor, M., & Phillips, J.K. (2007). Lack of functional expression of NMDA receptors in PC12 cells. *Neurotoxicology*, Vol.28, No.4, pp. 876-885

Fulda, S. (2010). Modulation of apoptosis by natural products for cancer therapy. *Planta Med*, Vol.76, No.11, pp. 1075-1079

Greene, L.A., & Tischler, A.S. (1976). Establishment of a noradrenergic clonal line of rat adrenal pheochromocytoma cells which respond to nerve growth factor. *Proc Natl Acad Sci U S A*, Vol.73, No.7, pp. 2424-2428

Gregory, C.D., & Pound, J.D. (2011). Cell death in the neighbourhood: direct microenvironmental effects of apoptosis in normal and neoplastic tissues. *J Pathol*, Vol.223, No.2, pp. 177-194

Jin, Z., & El-Deiry, W.S. (2005). Overview of cell death signaling pathways. *Cancer Biol Ther*, Vol.4, No.2, pp. 139-163

Karagiannis, A., Mikhailidis, D.P., Athyros, V.G., & Harsoulis, F. (2007). Pheochromocytoma: an update on genetics and management. *Endocr Relat Cancer*, Vol.14, No.4, pp. 935-956

Kondo, K., Obitsu, S., Ohta, S., Matsunami, K., Otsuka, H., & Teshima, R. (2010). Poly(ADP-ribose) polymerase (PARP)-1-independent apoptosis-inducing factor (AIF) release and cell death are induced by eleostearic acid and blocked by alpha-tocopherol and MEK inhibition. *J Biol Chem*, Vol.285, No.17, pp. 13079-13091

Lee, E., Williams, Z., Goodman, C.B., Oriaku, E.T., Harris, C., Thomas, M., & Soliman, K.F. (2006). Effects of NMDA receptor inhibition by phencyclidine on the neuronal differentiation of PC12 cells. *Neurotoxicology*, Vol.27, No.4, pp. 558-566

Molatore, S., Liyanarachchi, S., Irmler, M., Perren, A., Mannelli, M., Ercolino, T., Beuschlein, F., Jarzab, B., Wloch, J., Ziaja, J., Zoubaa, S., Neff, F., Beckers, J., Hofler, H., Atkinson, M.J., & Pellegata, N.S. (2010). Pheochromocytoma in rats with multiple endocrine neoplasia (MENX) shares gene expression patterns with human pheochromocytoma. *Proc Natl Acad Sci U S A*, Vol.107, No.43, pp. 18493-18498

Ohta, S., Lai, E.W., Taniguchi, S., Tischler, A.S., Alesci, S., & Pacak, K. (2006). Animal models of pheochromocytoma including NIH initial experience. *Ann N Y Acad Sci*, Vol.1073, pp. 300-305

Petri, B.J., van Eijck, C.H., de Herder, W.W., Wagner, A., & de Krijger, R.R. (2009). Phaeochromocytomas and sympathetic paragangliomas. *Br J Surg*, Vol.96, No.12, pp. 1381-1392

Pfragner, R., Behmel, A., Smith, D.P., Ponder, B.A., Wirnsberger, G., Rinner, I., Porta, S., Henn, T., & Niederle, B. (1998). First continuous human pheochromocytoma cell line: KNA. Biological, cytogenetic and molecular characterization of KNA cells. *J Neurocytol*, Vol.27, No.3, pp. 175-186

Powers, J.F., Evinger, M.J., Tsokas, P., Bedri, S., Alroy, J., Shahsavari, M., & Tischler, A.S. (2000). Pheochromocytoma cell lines from heterozygous neurofibromatosis knockout mice. *Cell Tissue Res*, Vol.302, No.3, pp. 309-320

Pytlowany, M., Strosznajder, J.B., Jesko, H., Cakala, M., & Strosznajder, R.P. (2008). Molecular mechanism of PC12 cell death evoked by sodium nitroprusside, a nitric oxide donor. *Acta Biochim Pol*, Vol.55, No.2, pp. 339-347

Reuter, S., Gupta, S.C., Chaturvedi, M.M., & Aggarwal, B.B. (2010). Oxidative stress, inflammation, and cancer: how are they linked? *Free Radic Biol Med*, Vol.49, No.11, pp. 1603-1616

Shacka, J.J., Sahawneh, M.A., Gonzalez, J.D., Ye, Y.Z., D'Alessandro, T.L., & Estevez, A.G. (2006). Two distinct signaling pathways regulate peroxynitrite-induced apoptosis in PC12 cells. *Cell Death Differ*, Vol.13, No.9, pp. 1506-1514

Terasawa, K., Ichimura, A., Sato, F., Shimizu, K., & Tsujimoto, G. (2009). Sustained activation of ERK1/2 by NGF induces microRNA-221 and 222 in PC12 cells. *Febs J*, Vol.276, No.12, pp. 3269-3276

Tischler, A.S., Powers, J.F., & Alroy, J. (2004). Animal models of pheochromocytoma. *Histol Histopathol*, Vol.19, No.3, pp. 883-895

Venihaki, M., Gravanis, A., & Margioris, A.N. (1998). KAT45 human pheochromocytoma cell line. A new model for the in vitro study of neuro-immuno-hormonal interactions. *Ann N Y Acad Sci*, Vol.840, pp. 425-433

Zangemeister-Wittke, U., & Simon, H.U. (2001). Apoptosis--regulation and clinical implications. *Cell Death Differ*, Vol.8, No.5, pp. 537-544

Ziegler, C.G., Brown, J.W., Schally, A.V., Erler, A., Gebauer, L., Treszl, A., Young, L., Fishman, L.M., Engel, J.B., Willenberg, H.S., Petersenn, S., Eisenhofer, G., Ehrhart-Bornstein, M., & Bornstein, S.R. (2009). Expression of neuropeptide hormone receptors in human adrenal tumors and cell lines: antiproliferative effects of peptide analogues. *Proc Natl Acad Sci U S A*, Vol.106, No.37, pp. 15879-15884

Part 4

Clinical Presentation

7

Headache in Pheochromocytoma

Masahiko Watanabe
Department of Neurology,
University of Tsukuba
Japan

1. Introduction

Two motives have combined to make me write a paper on headache in patients with pheochromocytoma. First, I would like to contribute to the clinical practices of both endocrinological clinicians who are working with patients with pheochromocytoma and neurologists who are performing headache consultations by elucidating the clinical characteristics of headache in patients with pheochromocytoma. Second, I will discuss the stereotypy of current diagnostic criteria provided by "The international classification of headache disorders," 2nd edition (ICHDII)(1) by reviewing the literature concerning the mechanism of headache attributed to pheochromocytoma.

Pheochromocytoma is a rare tumor arising from the chromaffin tissue. Although it is well-known to produce catecholamine , the tumor is frequently disclosed incidentally by autopsy or adrenal imaging.(2)-(3) The representative clinical features are characterized by the pentad of symptoms known as the "5Hs", that is headache, hypertension, hyperglycemia, hypermetabolism, and hyperhydrosis. Among these symptoms, which are attributed to the overproduction of catecholamine by the tumor, headache is important for four reasons. First, it is one of the most frequent symptoms.(4)(5)(6)(7) Second, it is frequently the presenting symptom.(8) Third, it may be the only symptom.(9)(10) Fourth, it may be the presenting symptom of a life-threatening disease with a histopathologically confirmed tumor.(11)(7)

2. Clinical characteristics of headache attributed to pheochromocytoma

Paroxysmal headache occurs in 51-80% of patients with pheochromocytoma. The most characteristic feature of the headache is its rapid onset. It nearly always seems to reach its peak within minutes, sometimes within one minute (thunderclap headache).(10)(12-14) It usually occurs spontaneously, but recurrent severe headaches may occur after voiding in patients with bladder pheochromocytoma.(13, 15)

An important feature of the paroxysmal headache is its short duration. In 50% of patients it lasts for less than 15 minutes, and in 70% its duration is less than one hour.(4) However, in patients with migraine, it may last longer.(8)

The headache was nearly always bilateral, (8) affecting any part of the head. The occipital, nuchal-occipital, and frontal-occipital regions are the predominant locations.(4) The headache is generally described as throbbing, pulsating, or bursting in quality, and is moderately to very severe in intensity.(8) As in the other patients with pheochromocytoma, headaches are frequently associated with palpitation and perspiration. Other features include apprehension and/or anxiety, often with a sense of impending death, tremor, visual disturbances, abdominal or chest pain, nausea, vomiting, and occasionally paraesthesia. The face can blanch or flush during attack.

The headaches are sometimes worse when lying down and sometimes made worse by moving.(8) Stress maneuvers such as coughing, sneezing, bending, and straining commonly aggravate the pain.(4) Measurement of blood pressure before and after onset of the headache revealed a sudden increase in both systolic and diastolic blood pressure.(8)

3. Diagnosis of headache attributed to pheochromocytoma

Diagnostic cues are usually provided by additional symptoms attributed to sympathetic activation, such as diaphoresis, palpitation, apprehension, and/or anxiety. The diagnosis is established by the demonstration of increased excretion of catecholamines or catecholamine metabolites, and can usually be verified by analysis of a single 24-hour urine sample collected when the patient is hypertensive or symptomatic.

4. Differential diagnosis

The typical case with the full-blown syndrome (5Hs) is not difficult to diagnose, but in some cases of pheochromocytoma, the symptoms are very subtle or absent except for severe headache. The most important point is to include pheochromocytoma in the differential diagnosis of a case with episodic headache. Further, careful history taking with close attention to sympathetic autonomic features will guide physicians to the right path.

Development of radiology enables us to exclude most secondary headache disorders easily, but in all primary headaches and some secondary headaches, brain imaging studies reveal no changes. In the case of pheochromocytoma, normal brain imaging is not the end but the starting point for the differential diagnosis.

4.1 Cluster headache and other trigeminal autonomic cephalalgia

Among the primary headaches, cluster headache is most similar to pheochromocytoma headache. An episodic pattern of occurrence, sudden onset, rapid evolution, short duration, and severity characterize both headaches. However, cluster headache is strictly unilateral and has parasympathetic autonomic system features, while pheochromocytoma headache is usually bilateral and has sympathetic autonomic system features. In addition to the difference in autonomic features, its unilaterality is also characteristic of cluster headache. Pain is usually more localized to the orbital area in patients with cluster headache. If these two diseases are confounded, highly critical outcomes may follow. In one reported cases, for example, dihydroergotamine, an agent sometimes used to treat cluster headache, was administered errorneously to a patient with pheochromocytoma, causing a hypertensive crisis and posterior reversible encephalopathy syndrome.(16)

4.2 Migraine

Because migraine is one of the commonest headache disorders, it is always included in the differential diagnosis of headache disorders. Classical migraine with aura will be no diagnostic problem, but a bilateral episodic headache without aura, should be differentiated from other disorders, including pheochromocytoma. Particularly, if the history of headaches is short and their duration is brief, it will be a diagnostic challenge. Nausea is usually associated with both types of headache. Magnetic resonance imaging of the brain is useless in the differential diagnosis of these two. Careful history taking with particular attention to additional features, including scotoma, photophobia, and sympathetic autonomic symptoms reveals the correct diagnosis.

4.3 Thunderclap headache (TCH)

Thunderclap headache (TCH) is defined as a severe head pain with sudden onset, reaching its maximum intensity in less than 1 minute and lasting from 1 hour to 10 days. Subarachnoid hemorrhage is by far the most common and most dangerous cause of thunderclap headache, but numerous other diseases involving the vasculature of the central nervous system, such as ischemic stroke, cerebral venous thrombosis, cervical arterial dissection, acute hypertensive crisis, retroclival hematoma, pituitary apoplexy, and the non-vascular structures of the central nervous system, such as spontaneous intracranial hypotension, third ventricle colloid cyst, and intracranial infection are found on the list of the diseases to be excluded in the differential diagnosis. Therefore, TCH is a particularly important symptom in differential diagnosis by cranial imaging. However, it is also important to bear in mind that many other diseases associated with TCHs, such as pheochromocytoma(10, 12-14) and myocardial infarction, cannot be detected by cranial imaging and may have serious outcomes.

4.4 Tension-type headache (TTH)

Tension-type headache (TTH) is the most common type of primary headache, and its lifetime prevalence in the general population is estimated to be from 30% to 78%. TTH is subdivided into episodic and chronic subtypes. Episodic TTH is further subdivided into frequent and infrequent subtypes. Frequent episodic TTH may be a candidate for the diagnosis of pheochromocytoma. It is usually bilateral and non-throbbing in nature. The intensity of the headache is mild to moderate, and it is not aggravated by routine physical activity. It lacks nausea, vomiting, arterial hypertension, or other sympathetic autonomic features (palpitation, perspiration, pallor, tremor, or anxiety).

4.5 Headache attributed to arterial hypertension

Mild (140-159/90-99 mmHg) or moderate (160-179/100-109 mmHg) chronic arterial hypertension does not cause headache.(17) Ambulatory blood pressure monitoring in patients with mild to moderate hypertension has shown no convincing relationship between blood pressure fluctuations over a 24-hour period and the presence or absence of headache.(18) However, paroxysmal hypertension may cause headache. "Headache attributed to hypertensive crisis without hypertensive encephalopathy" is defined as a bilateral pulsating headache that may be precipitated by physical activity and associated with a hypertensive crisis. A hypertensive crisis is defined as a paroxysmal rise in systolic (to $\geqq$180 mmHg) and/or diastolic (to $\geqq$120 mmHg) blood pressure but without clinical features of hypertensive encephalopathy. Further, headache that develops during a hypertensive crisis should resolve within one hour after normalization of blood pressure.(1) The mechanism of this type of headache is not fully understood. Failure of baroreceptor reflexes (after carotid endarterectomy or subsequent to irradiation of the neck) is thought to be a one of the mechanisms. Although it shows no sympathetic autonomic features, the rest of the characterisics of this headache are quite similar to pheochromocytoma headache. Again, it is important to ask the patient about their present and past history of sympathetic autonomic symptoms (palpitation, perspiration, pallor, tremor, or anxiety) and neck surgery.

4.6 Intracranial pheochromocytoma

Brain metastases of pheochromocytoma are extremely rare, and intracranial lesions are the only sites of metastasis in patients with adrenal pheochromocytoma. Mercuri et al. reported a primary meningeal pheochromocytoma that presented with headache, vomitting, and arterial hypertension.(19) Laboratory studies revealed high plasma catecholamines (norepinephrine and epinephrine). The tumor was resected, and histopathological examination confirmed the diagnosis. Six years follow-up after surgery showed that the patient was neurologically intact with normalized blood pressure and catecholamine values. This case is a very rare exception in which cranial imaging study provided the crucial information to make a diagnosis of headache attributed to pheochromocytoma.

4.7 Spontaneous intracranial hemorrhage due to pheochromocytoma

Park et al. reported an 18-year-old man who presented with a sudden onset of headaches, followed by left hemianopsia.(20) He had experienced palpitations and chest discomfort during physical exertion for two years prior to admission. A brain CT scan showed intracerebral hemorrhage in the left frontoparietal area. Hypertension in the form of paroxysmal attacks led the authors to suspect pheochromocytoma. Evaluation of a 24-h urine specimen showed elevated vanillylmandelic acid and metanephrine levels. Abdominal CT demonstrated a para-aortic mass, and ^{131}I-metaiodobenzylguanidine (MIBG) scintigraphy showed high uptake in the same area. This case typically showed that cranial imaging is useless to make a correct diagnosis of headache caused by pheochromocytoma.

4.8 Pheochromocytoma crisis induced by glucocorticoids

Pheochromocytoma crisis (PC) is a rare life-threatening endocrineological emergency that may present spontaneously or can be elicited by triggers, including certain medications that trigger the release of catecholamines by tumors. Acute and rapidly progressive hemodynamic disturbances result from the actions of high quantities of catecholamines secreted by the tumor. Hypertensive crisis, cardiac ischemia, cardiogenic shock, and end-organ failure may occur. Some patients show headache concomitant with hypertension. Many drugs can cause adverse reactions in patients with pheochromocytoma, but we also have to keep in mind that a high-dose dexamethasone suppression test (DST) may precipitate PC in cases with incidental adrenal masses.(21)

5. Headache and hypertension

Recording of blood pressure before and after the onset of the headache revealed a sudden increase in both systolic and diastolic blood pressure.(8) Probably because of this single sign, the diagnostic criteria proposed in "The international classification of headache disorders, 2nd edition (ICHD-II)" included concomitant hypertension as a mandatory item for the diagnosis of headache attributed to pheochromocytoma.(1) However, in some patients, very high blood pressures were observed without concomitant headache.(8) In addition, observation of normal or low blood pressure in pheochromocytoma cases is not particularly rare,(22) and it is known that catecholamine concentrations in circulating blood are not well correlated with blood pressure. There were other cases in which hypertension was not observed despite confirmation of urinary cathecholamine metabolite elevation.(23)

6. Mechanism of headache in patients with pheochromocytoma

The mechanism of headache associated with pheochromocytoma is not fully understood. According to the International Classification of Headache Disorders; 2nd Edition (ICHDII), the diagnosis of headache attributed to pheochromocytoma is established by fulfillment of the following two conditions. First, headache develops concomitantly with an abrupt rise in blood pressure. Second, headache resolves or markedly improves within 1 hour of normalization of blood pressure. However, not a small number of patients who were demonstrated to have pheochromocytoma by biochemical or radiological examination and/or histopathological findings of their surgical specimens showed typical headache without hypertension.(14, 23) Therefore, hypertension is not the only factor in headache pathogenesis.(24)

6.1 Catecholamines and headache

The human cerebral circulation is innervated by sympathetic nerves. The sympathetic system contains the transmitters noradrenaline, neuropeptide Y (NPY), and possibly adenosinetriphosphate (ATP) and is a vasoconstrictor pathway.(25) The cranial vessels are also innervated by the trigeminal nerve. This system is marked by the presence of calcitonin gene-related peptide (CGRP), substance P, and neurokinin A. It is a vasodilator pathway(26) via antidromic release upon activation as well as having a primary involvement in sensory function.(27)

It is hardly possible to connect throbbing headache with the direct action of the strong vasopressor, noradrenalin, which usually causes hypertension in patients with pheochromocytoma. Lance et al. studied the relationship between the main subtype of catecholamine produced by the pheochromocytoma and clinical symptoms of patients. They concluded that the presence or absence of headache or quality of the headache did not bear any relationship to the ratio of norepinephrine to epinephrine secreted.(8) Intravenous infusion of norepinephrine into a patient susceptible to migraine at a sufficient concentration to raise the systolic blood pressure 10 to 40 mmHg is not sufficient to produce headache. Wolff et al. administered such infusions on 116 occasions to 35 patients with vascular headaches of the migraine type, with abolition or reduction in intensity of headache in 93 instances. In these cases, the diameter of the temporal artery and the amplitude of its pulse wave were observed to diminish as the headache abated.

6.2 Neuropeptides and headache

It seems quite plausible that strong vasodilator peptides produced by pheochromocytoma, such as adrenomedullin(28) and CGRP(23) can cause episodic vascular headaches characterized by throbbing in patients with pheochromocytoma. The headache-inducing property of CGRP has been studied in one double-blind controlled trial.(29) The headache was pulsating in quality and resolved within 1 hour after ingestion of CGRP. In addition, a recent study showed that a CGRP antagonist is effective in the acute treatment of migraine.(30) To elucidate a possible role of CGRP in the pathological mechanism of pheochromocytoma headache, a trial using a CGRP antagonist in patients with pheochromocytoma headache should be performed.

7. Conclusion

It is very important to understand the characteristics of the headache attributed to pheochromocytoma because it is one of the most frequent symptoms of a disease that is frequently neglected clinically. It is also important to consider during headache consultation because both neurological and radiological examinations of the brain will provide little information for the correct diagnosis.

The mechanism of the headache in patients with pheochromocytoma is not fully understood. In addition to the arterial hypertension, vasodilator peptides produced by the tumor may play important roles.

8. References

[1] Headache Classification Subcommittee of the International Headache Society. The international classification of headache disorders: 2nd edition. Cephalalgia. 2004;24 Suppl 1:9-160.

[2] Kopetschke R, Slisko M, Kilisli A, Tuschy U, Wallaschofski H, Fassnacht M, et al. Frequent incidental discovery of phaeochromocytoma: Data from a german cohort of 201 phaeochromocytoma. Eur J Endocrinol. 2009 Aug;161(2):355-61.

[3] Manger WM. The protean manifestations of pheochromocytoma. Horm Metab Res. 2009 Sep;41(9):658-63.

[4] Thomas JE, Rooke ED, Kvale WF. The neurologist's experience with pheochromocytoma. A review of 100 cases. JAMA. 1966 Sep 5;197(10):754-8.

[5] Loh KC, Shlossberg AH, Abbott EC, Salisbury SR, Tan MH. Phaeochromocytoma: A ten-year survey. QJM. 1997 Jan;90(1):51-60.

[6] Mannelli M, Ianni L, Cilotti A, Conti A. Pheochromocytoma in italy: A multicentric retrospective study. Eur J Endocrinol. 1999 Dec;141(6):619-24.

[7] Manger WM, Gifford RW. Pheochromocytoma. J Clin Hypertens (Greenwich). 2002 Jan-Feb;4(1):62-72.

[8] Lance JW, Hinterberger H. Symptoms of pheochromocytoma, with particular reference to headache, correlated with catecholamine production. Arch Neurol. 1976 Apr;33(4):281-8.

[9] Udayakumar N, Sivaprakash S, Chandrasekaran M. Headache as the only sign of pheochromocytoma: An analysis. Indian J Med Sci. 2007 Nov;61(11):611-3.

[10] Sanyal K, Fletcher S. Headache as a sign of phaeochromocytoma. Emerg Med J. 2009 Jan;26(1):71.

[11] Verrijcken A, Sciot R, Dubois CL. From trivial headache to life-threatening disease. Int J Cardiol. 2011 Jan 7;146(1):e7-9.

[12] Heo YE, Kwon HM, Nam HW. Thunderclap headache as an initial manifestation of phaeochromocytoma. Cephalalgia. 2009 Mar;29(3):388-90.

[13] Im SH, Kim NH. Thunderclap headache after micturition in bladder pheochromocytoma. Headache. 2008 Jun;48(6):965-7.
[14] Watanabe M, Takahashi A, Shimano H, Hara H, Sugita S, Nakamagoe K, et al. Thunderclap headache without hypertension in a patient with pheochromocytoma. J Headache Pain. 2010 Oct;11(5):441-4.
[15] Mou JW, Lee KH, Tam YH, Cheung ST, Chan KW, Thakre A. Urinary bladder pheochromocytoma, an extremely rare tumor in children: Case report and review of the literature. Pediatr Surg Int. 2008 Apr;24(4):479-80.
[16] Kelley BJ, Samples S, Kunkel R. PRES following administration of DHE in a patient with unsuspected pheochromocytoma. Headache. 2008 Sep;48(8):1237-9.
[17] Kruszewski P, Bieniaszewski L, Neubauer J, Krupa-Wojciechowska B. Headache in patients with mild to moderate hypertension is generally not associated with simultaneous blood pressure elevation. J Hypertens. 2000 Apr;18(4):437-44.
[18] Gus M, Fuchs FD, Pimentel M, Rosa D, Melo AG, Moreira LB. Behavior of ambulatory blood pressure surrounding episodes of headache in mildly hypertensive patients. Arch Intern Med. 2001 Jan 22;161(2):252-5.
[19] Mercuri S, Gazzeri R, Galarza M, Esposito S, Giordano M. Primary meningeal pheochromocytoma: Case report. J Neurooncol. 2005 Jun;73(2):169-72.
[20] Park SK, Lee JK, Joo SP, Kim TS, Kim JH, Kim SH, et al. Spontaneous intracerebral haemorrhage caused by extra-adrenal phaeochromocytoma. J Clin Neurosci. 2006 Apr;13(3):388-90.
[21] Rosas AL, Kasperlik-Zaluska AA, Papierska L, Bass BL, Pacak K, Eisenhofer G. Pheochromocytoma crisis induced by glucocorticoids: A report of four cases and review of the literature. Eur J Endocrinol. 2008 Mar;158(3):423-9.
[22] Bravo EL, Tarazi RC, Gifford RW, Stewart BH. Circulating and urinary catecholamines in pheochromocytoma. diagnostic and pathophysiologic implications. N Engl J Med. 1979 Sep 27;301(13):682-6.
[23] Agarwal A, Gupta S, Mishra AK, Singh N, Mishra SK. Normotensive pheochromocytoma: Institutional experience. World J Surg. 2005 Sep;29(9):1185-8.
[24] Piovesan EJ, Moeller L, Piovesan LM, Werneck LC, de Carvalho JL. Headache in patients with pheochromocytoma. influence of arterial hypertension. Arq Neuropsiquiatr. 1998 Jun;56(2):255-7.
[25] Edvinsson L, Owman C, Sjoberg NO. Autonomic nerves, mast cells, and amine receptors in human brain vessels. A histochemical and pharmacological study. Brain Res. 1976 Oct 22;115(3):377-93.
[26] Hong KW, Yoo SE, Yu SS, Lee JY, Rhim BY. Pharmacological coupling and functional role for CGRP receptors in the vasodilation of rat pial arterioles. Am J Physiol. 1996 Jan;270(1 Pt 2):H317-23.
[27] McCulloch J, Uddman R, Kingman TA, Edvinsson L. Calcitonin gene-related peptide: Functional role in cerebrovascular regulation. Proc Natl Acad Sci U S A. 1986 Aug;83(15):5731-5.
[28] Kitamura K, Kangawa K, Kawamoto M, Ichiki Y, Nakamura S, Matsuo H, et al. Adrenomedullin: A novel hypotensive peptide isolated from human pheochromocytoma. Biochem Biophys Res Commun. 1993 Apr 30;192(2):553-60.

[29] Lassen LH, Haderslev PA, Jacobsen VB, Iversen HK, Sperling B, Olesen J. CGRP may play a causative role in migraine. Cephalalgia. 2002 Feb;22(1):54-61.

[30] Olesen J, Diener HC, Husstedt IW, Goadsby PJ, Hall D, Meier U, et al. Calcitonin gene-related peptide receptor antagonist BIBN 4096 BS for the acute treatment of migraine. N Engl J Med. 2004 Mar 11;350(11):1104-10.

8

Primary Cardiac Pheochromocytoma (Paraganglioma)

Iskander Al-Githmi
Division of Cardiothoracic Surgery
Faculty of Medicine, King Abdulaziz University
Jeddah
Saudi Arabia

1. Introduction

Pheochromocytomas are catecholamine-producing neuroendocrine tumors arise from primitive neural crest cells. About 90% of these tumors occur as solitary benign tumors of the adrenal medulla, where majority of chromaffin cells are concentrated. Only ten percent originates from extra-adrenal sites with the organ of Zukerkandal (paraganglia along abdominal aorta) being the most common. Chromaffin cells can also be found in the wall of blood vessels, along the aorta, prostate, urinary bladder and ovaries. Primary cardiac pheochromocytomas are extremely rare, occurring in only 0.001% to 0.03% of several reported autopsy series. Most of these tumors are found in the left atrium, possibly explained by close proximity of paraganglionic cell nest to the left atrium. Primary cardiac pheochromocytoms produce large amount of catecholamine, primarily norepinephrine and less frequently epinephrine.

2. Pathophysiology and pathology

Cardiac pheochromocytomas occur at any age, but mostly in the fourth and fifth decades of live. They are extremely vascular, their blood supply exclusively derived from coronary circulation. These tumors are usually functional, producing excessive amount of catecholamines, primarily secrete norepinephrine, which is a potent vasoconstrictor and raises the peripheral vascular resistance. Therefore, systolic blood pressure rises, but diastolic blood pressure may fall. It has very minimal, if any, direct effect on the heart, actually, cardiac output may fall reflexly as a result of an increase in the blood pressure. Cardiac pheochromcytoma arise from branchiomeric (coronary, pulmonary or aortopulmonary) paraganglia or visceral autonomic (atrium or interatrial septum) paraganglia. Often, they are dark red-brownish, soft, fleshy and highly vascular non encapsulated tumors that found under the aorta and pulmonary artery in association with left atrium (Figure 1). They can extend into the atrio-ventricular groove and the coronary arteries. Malignant changes are present in 10% of catecholamine-secreting tumors as defined by presence of metastasis or local tissue invasion. Cardiac pheochromocytomas appear more invasive and difficult to "shell out", unlike benign adrenal pheochromocytomas.

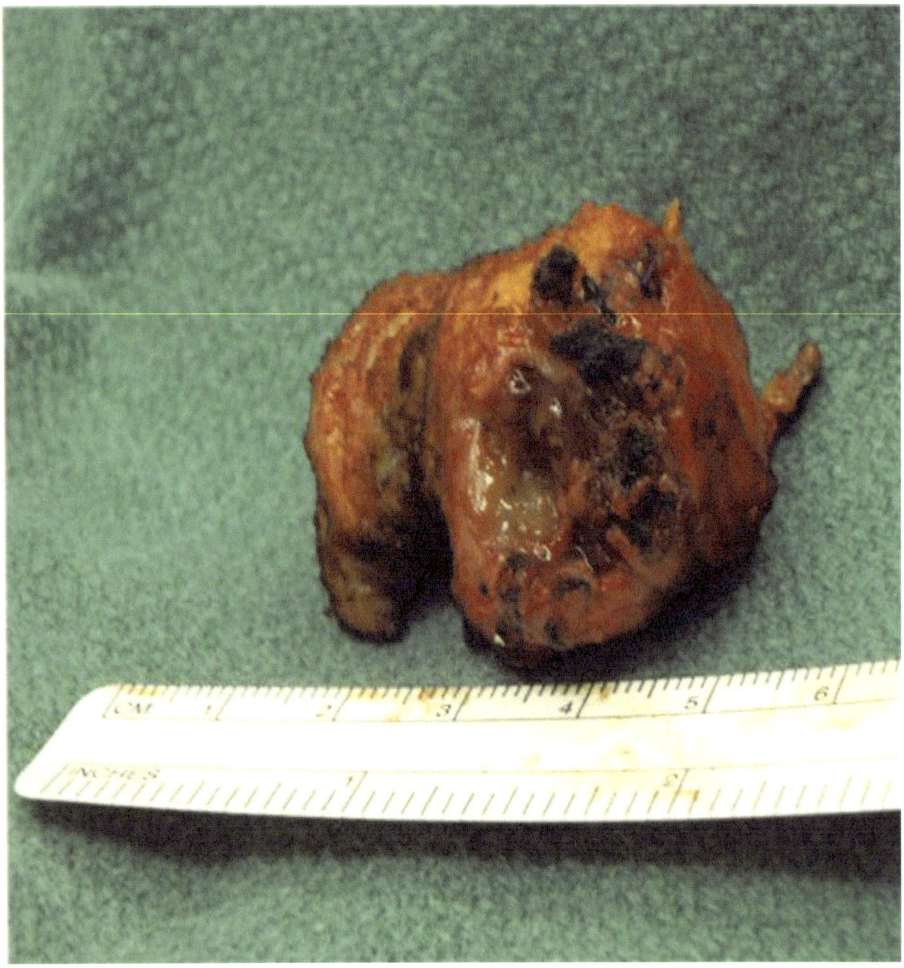

Fig. 1. Resected cardiac pheochromocytoma.

3. Clinical manifestations

The clinical manifestation of cardiac pheochromocytoma can be related to catecholamine secretion, size of the tumor and competition for blood supply with normal myocardium. Headache, excess sweating, flushing and palpitation are the usual symptoms of cardiac pheochromocytomas. Sustained, labile, or paroxysmal hypertension is typically present in almost all patients with cardiac pheochromocytomas as a result of excess circulating catecholamines. These tumors can cause angina chest pain as it competes with normal myocardium for coronary blood supply. Occasionally seizures occur and very rarely intense mesenteric artery vasoconstriction may cause ischemic enterocolitis with severe abdominal pain. However clinical manifestations of cardiac pheochromocytomas are less dramatic compared to adrenal pheochromocytoma. We reported a case presenting with angina chest pain and the tumor received dual blood supply from both right and left coronary arteries and had undergone complete surgical excision utilizing cardiopulmonary bypass (Figure 3, 4).

4. Diagnosis

Clinical suspicion is raised in cases of resistant hypertension particularly in patients with family history of pheochromocytoma. Quantification of the plasma or urinary catecholamine metabolite metanephrine is the most sensitive test for the diagnosis (sensitivity 99%, specificity 81%) in one study that compared biochemical markers in detection of catecholamine-secreting tumors. In addition, contrasted enhanced computed tomography of the abdomen is indicated to rule out adrenal gland involvement. Anatomic localization of cardiac pheochromocytomas can be made with high speed dynamic computed tomography with intravenous contrast bolus administration (Figure 2). Magnetic resonance imaging has been found to be more sensitive in the localization of extra-adrenal pheochromocytoma based on greater resolution and sensitivity for soft tissue. Pheochromocytomas demonstrate a hyper-intense signal on T2-weighted images and typically iso-hypo-intense relative to myocardium on T1-weighted images. Presence of peripheral rim enhancement on late gadolinium enhancement (LGE) indicates vascularity of cardiac pheochromocytomas distinguishing them from a vascular cardiac mass such as cardiac thrombi and lipoma. Total body 123-iodine-iodobenzylguanidine (MIBG) scintigraphy scan is well established for preoperative localization of cardiac pheochromocytoma and has also been found to be of use in locating other neural-endocrine tumors and search for metastatic disease. A recent study, Indium–Octereotide uptake scan has been described in cardiac pheochromocytoma, but its clinical significance is not well established. Coronary angiography is useful in judging local excision of the disease, coronary artery involvement and screening for atherosclerotic disease in these patients with hypertension.

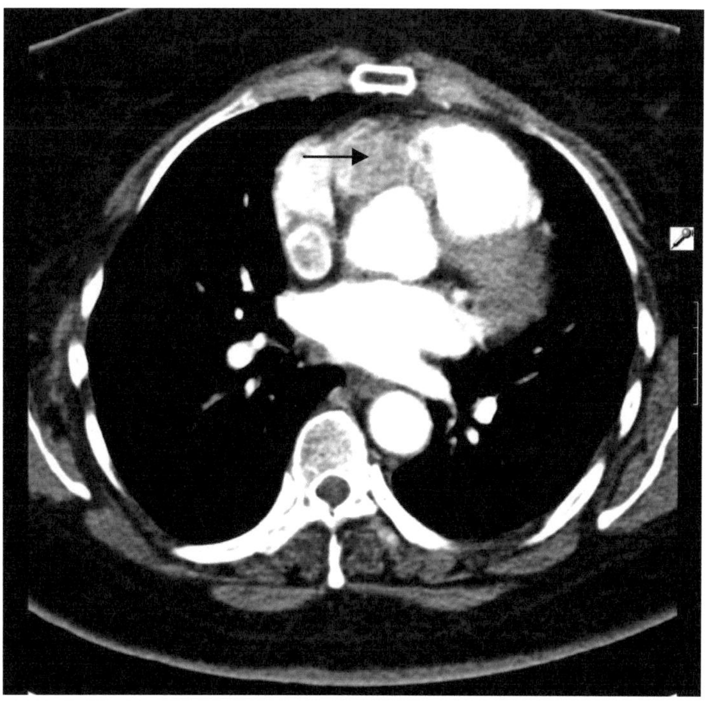

Fig. 2. Computed tomography scan of chest demonstrating a mass overlay the aortic root and extended through right ventricular muscle fibers (arrow).

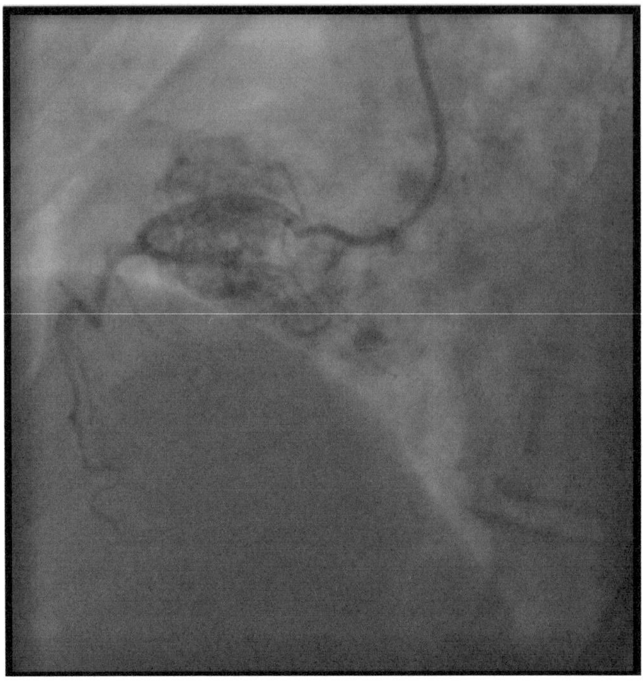

Fig. 3. Coronary angiogram: showing right coronary artery tumor blush.

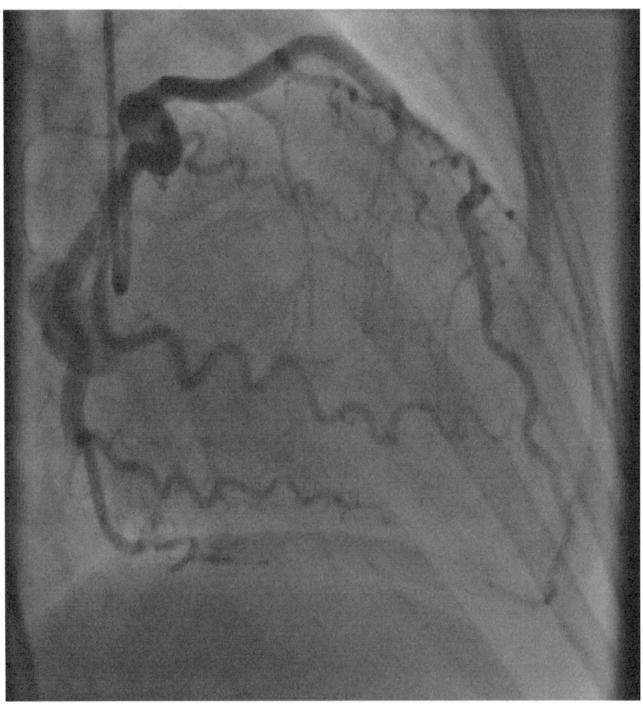

Fig. 4. Coronary angiogram: showing left circumflex coronary arteries tumor blush.

5. Management

Complete Surgical resection with adequate disease-free margins and reconstruction with pericardial or synthetic patch is the gold standard treatment for primary cardiac pheochromocytomas, but this can be technically difficult and is complicated by the position and extension of the tumor. These include pheochromocytoma extension into atrioventricular groove, direct coronary artery involvement and extension into the left ventricle. In these patients, resection with adequate margin carries high mortality and morbidity as a result of fatal hemorrhage and myocardial infarction. In this group of patients cardiac transplantation is the best treatment option provided distant metastasis has been excluded. Adequate preoperative preparation with alpha and beta adrenergic blockers and total cardiopulmonary bypass with cardioplegic arrest should be instituted to isolate the heart from systemic circulation before manipulation of the tumor. However, in all patients, life-long surveillance for recurrence should be performed with regular follow-up employing biochemical testing for fractionated metanephrines and imaging techniques such as 123-iodine-iodobenzylguanidine (MIBG) and computed tomography scans when appropriate.

6. Conclusion

Primary cardiac pheochromocytomas are very rare tumor of the heart. The multimodality imaging studies in assessing cardiac tumor are important in planning surgical strategy. Complete resection of cardiac pheochromocytoma with adequate disease free margin is the standard treatment which safely performed using cardiopulmonary bypass. Long-term surveillance is warranted for tumor recurrence.

7. Acknowledgment

The author expresses his gratitude to his wife Dr. Nadia Batawil for her outstanding support.

8. References

Manger WA. 2006 An overview of pheochromocytoma, history current concepts, vagaries and diagnostic challenges Ann N Y Acad Sci, 1073, 1-20.

Jeevandam V, Oz MC, Shapiro B, Barr MI, Marboe C, Rose EA. 1995 Surgical management of cardiac pheochromocytoma. Resection versus transplantation. Ann Surg, 221, 415-9.

Lin JC, Palafox BA, Jackson HA, Cohen AJ, Gazzaniga AB. 1999 Cardiac pheochromocytoma resectionafter diagnosis by 111-Indium octreotide scan. Ann Thorac Surg, 67, 555-8.

Al-Githmi IS, Baslaim GM, Batawil NA. 2010 Primary cardiac paraganglioma with dual coronary blood supply presenting with angina chest pain. Can J Cardiol, 26(7):278-279.

Sheehy N, Kulke MH, Abbeele AD. 2008 F-18 FDG/PET in the diagnosis and management of a pericardiac paraganglioma. Clin Nucl Med, 33, 545-6.

Lupinski RW, Shankar S, Agasthian T, Lim CH, Mancer K. 2004 Primary cardiac pheochromocytoma. Ann Thorac Surg, 78, e43-4.

Kennelly R, Aziz R, Toner M, Young V. 2008 Right atrial paraganglioma: an unusual primary cardiac tumor. Eur J Cardiothorac Surg, 33, 1150-2.

Shapiro B, 1993 Imaging of catecholamine-secreting tumors: uses of MIBG in diagnosis and treatment. Bailliere's Clinical Endocrinology and Metabolism, 7, 491-507.

Okum EJ, Henry D, Kasirajan V, DeAnda A, 2005 Cardiac pheochromocytoma. J Thorac Cardiovasc Surg, 129, 674-675.

Sawka AM, Young Jr Schaff HV, 2001 Cardiac phaeochromocytoma presenting with severe hypertension and chest pain, Clinical Endocrinology, 54, 689-692.

Brown ML, Zayas GE, Abel MD, Young WF Jr, Schaff HV, 2008 Mediastinal paragangliomas: the Mayo clinic experience, Ann Thorac Surg, 86, 946-51.

Part 5

Diagnosis

9

Diagnosis: Laboratorial Investigation and Imaging Methods

José Fernando Vilela-Martin and Luciana Neves Cosenso-Martin
State Medical School of São José do Rio Preto (FAMERP), São Paulo, Brazil

1. Introduction

Pheochromocytomas and paragangliomas are rare catechomine-producing tumors. Pheochromocytoma is a chromaffin tumor originating in the adrenal medulla and paraganglioma is originating in the sympathetic and parasympathetic portions of the autonomic nervous system paraganglia. The patients' symptoms are variable according the tumor secretion of norepinephrine (NE), epinephrine (E) or dopamine into the circulation. Patients with tumors predominantly secrete norepinephrine present with severe and refractory hypertension to conventional treatment. Patients with predominantly epinephrine and dopamine-secreting tumors present with episodic symptoms such as tachycardia with palpitations, panic attacks and feelings of doom.

1.1 Multiple Endocrine Neoplasia syndromes (MEN)

MEN 1 is a rare autosomal dominant disease that consists of tumors of the parathyroid glands, pancreatic islets (insulinomas) and anterior pituitary. Pheochromocytoma is not a feature in this syndrome.

MEN 2 is an autosomal dominant syndrome with three recognized sub-types: MEN 2A, B and C. In MEN 2A (Sipple's syndrome), medullary thyroid carcinoma is associated with pheochromocytoma and hyperparathyroidism. Pheochromocytoma is frequently bilateral and the diagnosis is later than medullary carcinoma. Patients who have been treated for medullary carcinoma should be screened for pheochromocytoma.

2. Epidemiology

The prevalence of pheochromocytoma is not precisely known. However, the incidence is about 1-2 per 100,000 adults per year according study in Minnesota (Beard et al., 1983). In countries other than United States, a lesser incidence has been noted about 2 to 8 cases per million inhabitants per year (Stenström & Svärdsudd, 1986). In a large series of patients screened biochemically for suspicion of pheochromocytoma, the incidence has been described to be as high as 1.9%. There was no difference between men and women (Smythe et al., 1992). Recently, a clinical review described the incidence between 2 and 8 cases per million per year in the United States (Golden et al., 2009). In an autopsy series described by McNeil et al. one pheochromocytoma occurred per 2301 autopsies (McNeil et al., 2000). With the routine use of computerized tomography (CT) for abdominal complaints, it is likely that more tumors will be discovered. The tumor is discovered incidentally in approximately 10% of patients during CT or magnetic resonance imaging (MRI) of the abdomen for unrelated symptoms (Kudva et al., 2003). However, recently others authors reported a 30% rate of incidentally discovered pheochromocytomas in their cohort of patients (Kopetschke et al., 2009; Shen et al., 2010). Pheochromocytoma is present in 0.1% to 1% of patients with hypertension (Omura et al., 2004)

Approximately 10% of adrenal pheochromocytomas and 30% of paragangliomas are considered malignant (Suh et al., 2009). 70% to 80% of pheochromocytomas occur sporadically. The familial syndromes that may present with pheochromocytoma include multiple endocrine neoplasia type 2 (NEM 2), von Hippel-Lindau syndrome, Osler-Weber-Rendu syndrome, and neurofibromatosis syndrome type 1 (Guerrero et al., 2009). The peak incidence occurs in the third to fifth decades of life and the average age at diagnosis is 43.9 years in sporadic cases (Neumann et al., 2002). However, the familial syndromes include younger patients (24.9 years), extra-adrenal and multiple tumors and the hypertension is persistent (Perel et al., 1997). Some authors studied genetic screening in pheochromocytoma and found younger patients with familial syndromes in their cohorts (Manelli et al., 2009; Cascon et al., 2009).

Pheochromocytoma was the most frequent indication for adrenalectomy (23.2%) noted by Villar (Villar et al., 2010).

The 10% rule is no longer applied. The ectopic pheochromocytoma is more prevalent than 10% (Madani et al., 2007). Extra-adrenal tumors are extra-adrenal paragangliomas and the majority is located in the head and neck area (69%), followed by intra-abdominal (22%) and intrathoracic locations (10%) (Van Der Horst-Schrivers et al., 2010). The periaortic, pericaval regions and Zuckerkandl's were the commonest sites of abdominal paragangliomas (Erickson et al., 2001).

3. Pathophysiology

3.1 The sympathetic nervous system (SNS)

The hypertension of pheochromocytoma has been thought to result solely from the action of circulating catecholamines on cardiovascular adrenergic receptors. However, according to the studies of Bravo *et al.*, blood pressure demonstrates no correlation with circulating catecholamines (Bravo et al., 1979). Bravo and collaborators related that sympathetic reflexes are intact, and blood pressure and heart rate are significantly reduced by clonidine despite maintained high circulating catecholamine (Bravo et al., 1982).

In pheochromocytoma patients, the SNS activity is enhanced and maintains the elevated blood pressure by the catecholamine-induced hypertension. The paradoxical elevation of sympathetic activity during elevation of circulating catecholamine is postulated to be due three mechanisms: 1) loading of sympathetic vesicles with catecholamine, presumably reflecting a loading of noradrenergic terminal vesicles with neurotransmitter; 2) increased sympathetic neuronal impulse frequency; and 3) a selective desensitization of presynaptic α_2 -adrenergic receptors. These receptors inhibit release of neuronal NE. Thus, selective desensitization results in enhanced release of neuronal NE during nerve stimulation.

The hypertensive crisis could be produced by any direct or reflexly mediated stimulus to the SNS, because of the enhanced SNS activity and excessive stores of NE in sympathetic nerve terminals (Bravo & Tagle, 2003).

3.2 The neurohumoral agents

Angiotensin II has no direct role in pheochromocytoma, because the administration of clonidine reduces arterial blood pressure without significantly decreasing plasma renin activity (Bravo et al., 1982). Neuropeptide Y (NPY) levels are increased in plasma and in tumors of patients with pheochromocytoma (deS Senanayake et al., 1995; Lundberg et al., 1986). NPY increases coronary and peripheral and vascular resistance independently of α-adrenergic mechanisms by interacting with vascular G protein-coupled receptors (O'Hare & Schwartz, 1989; Lundberg et al., 1982). The hypertensive episodes that occur in pheochromocytoma patients receiving α-blockade might be due the NPY release by the pheochromocytoma.

3.3 Hemodynamic characteristics

Pheochromocytoma patients have hemodynamic features similar to patients with essential hypertension. Thus, increased peripheral vascular resistance seems to be primarily responsible for maintenance of hypertension (Bravo & Tagle, 2003).

4. Diagnosis

Before discussing the role of laboratory diagnosis and research of imaging methods would be interesting to present the patient with symptoms of pheochromocytoma and the reasons would lead to further investigation. The table 1 shows the main points of clinical presentation for screening of pheochromocytoma. In addition, the table 2 shows the main differential diagnosis (Young & Sheps, 2008).

Episodic symptoms of headaches, tachycardia, and diaphoresis
Remember the five "H" characterizing pheochromocytoma: hypertension, hyperglycemia, hypermetabolism, hyperhidrosis and headache
Family history of pheochromocytoma or a MEN syndrome, VHL, or neurofibromatosis type 1
Incidental adrenal or abdominal masses
Unexplained paroxysms of tachyarrhythmias, bradyarrhythmias and / or hypertension during intubation, induction of anesthesia, parturition, or prolonged and unexplained hypotension after an operation
Adverse cardiovascular responses to ingestion, inhalation or injection of certain drugs (anesthetic agents, histamine, glucagons, naloxone, antidopaminergic agents, tricyclic antidepressants)
Attacks occurring during exertion, turning the torso, coitus, or micturition.

Table 1. Patients for screening of pheochromocytoma.

Endocrine • Thyrotoxicosis • Primary hypogonadism (e.g, menopausal syndrome) • Pancreatite tumors (e.g., insulinoma) • Medullary thyroid carcinoma • "Hyperadrenergic" spells
Cardiovascular • Essential hypertension, labile • Angina and cardiovascular deconditioning • Pulmonary edema • Dilated cardiomyopathy • Syncope • Orthostatic hypotension • Paroxysmal cardiac arrhythmia • Aortic dissection • Renovascular hypertension
Psychological • Anxiety and panic attacks • Somatization disorder • Hyperventilation • Factitious (e.g., drugs, Valsalva)
Pharmacologic • Withdrawal of adrenergic-inhibiting medication (e.g, clonidine) • Monoamine oxidase inhibitor treatment and concomitante ingestion of tyramine or a decongestant • Sympathomimetic ingestion • Ilicit drug ingestion (e.g, cocaine, phencyclidine, lysergic acid) • Acrodynia (Mercury poisoning) • Vancomycin (red man syndrome)
Neurologic • Baroreflex failure • Postural orthostatic tachycardia syndrome • Autonomic neuropathy • Migraine headache • Diencephalic epilepsy (autonomic seizures) • Cerebral infarction • Cerebrovascular insufficiency
Miscellaneous • Mastocytosis (systemic or activation disorder) • Carcinoid syndrome • Recurrent idiopathic anaphylaxis • Unexplained flushing spells

Table 2. Differential diagnosis of pheochromocytoma.

Approximately 50% of pheochromocytomas produce excessive amounts E and NE and the other 50% predominantely produce NE. Sympathetic paragangliomas produce mainly NE, frequently dopamine, and never E (Eisenhofer et al., 2003).
Measurements of fractionated metanephrines in urine and in plasma or both are the initial testing for pheochromocytoma (Lenders et al., 2002) and no single analysis can achieve 100% accuracy for pheochromocytoma diagnosis.
When the presence of a pheochromocytoma appears likely but with equivocal biochemical testing, a clonidine test is recommended to distinguish true from false positives results (Eisenhofer et al., 2003).
Levels of normetanephrine, metanephrine, or both metabolites are increased in almost all patients with pheochromocytoma. However, in small or microscopic tumors (<1 cm) producing small amounts of catecholamines, the levels of normetanephrine and metanephrine might be normal (Eisenhofer et al., 1999; Lenders et al., 2002). If there is a hereditary predisposition or a previous history for pheochromocytoma, a testing at a later date remains mandatory. False-negative results also could include patients with pheochromocytoma that do not produce NE or E, a more rare exception (Sawka et al., 2003).

4.1 Plasma metanephrines

Normal plasma levels of normetanephrine and metanephrine exclude pheochromocytoma, and no immediate testing for the tumor should be necessary. Thus, measurements of plasma free metanephrines eliminate false-negative in the diagnosis of pheochromocytoma. In contrast, false-positive results remain a common problem, potentially time-consuming and expensive for follow-up. Plasma free metanephrines sensitivity is 99%, followed closely by urinary fractionated metanephrines at 97% (Lenders et al., 2002). The blood sample should be obtained in the supine position. The technique involves the determination of free metanephrines in plasma by high-performance liquid chromatography (HPLC). An elevation of at least four times the upper reference intervals is associated with nearly a 100% probability of pheochromocytoma or sympathetic paraganglioma (Lenders et al., 2005). Elevated catecholamine and metanephrine levels by one to three times the upper limits of normality are usually due to various medications or physiological responses. For tests of plasma free metanephrines the specificity is 89% (Bravo & Tagle, 2003).
False-positive results include medical conditions, medications, inappropriate sampling conditions, and diet. An overnight fast and resting supine before blood sampling minimize the problem. Phenoxybenzamine and tricyclic antidepressants accounted for up to 45% of false-positive elevations of plasma or urinary norepinephrine and normetanephrine (Eisenhofer et al., 2003). However, selective serotonin reuptake inhibitors may provide an alternative medication because they are not a cause of false-positive results.
Phenoxybenzamine is a nonspecific α-adrenoreceptor blocker, causing norepinephrine and normetanephrine elevation by attenuating α_2-adrenoreceptor-mediated feedback inhibition of norepinephrine release, possibly combined with reflexive sympathetic activation. Thus, this drug should be avoided until biochemical testing is complete. Alternative medications for blood pressure control may include calcium channel blockers and selective α_1-adrenoreceptor blockers such as doxazosin and prazosin. Non-selective α-adrenoreceptor blockers were associated with 60% of all false-positive elevations of plasma metanephrine. Nevertheless, the false-positive rate was not high (12.5%). Only if an equivocal result has been obtained, it is necessary repeat testing after withdrawing these medications.

4.2 Urinary free catecholamines and metabolites

Urinary free NE and E and two major metabolites of the catecholamines, metanephrines (normetanephrines and metanephrines) and vanillylmandelic acid (VMA) are relatively easy to perform and are usually readly available. A diagnosis can be confirmed or excluded on the basis of properly collected 24h urine samples (Mannelli, 1989). In MEN syndromes, either 24-h urinary excretion or the calculated ratio of E to NE is a very sensitive screening test (Gagel et al, 1988). The sensitivity of the tests used to detect pheochromocytoma is as follows: urinary NE 86%, urinary E 33%, urinary VMA 64%, plasma NE 58%, and plasma E 33%. Among all tests for pheochromocytoma, the higher specificities are 95 % for test of urinary VMA and 93% for test of urinary total metanephrines (Bravo & Tagle, 2003). The table 3 shows the sensitivity and specificity values of diagnostic tests.

	Sensitivity %		**Specificity %**	
	Hereditary	Sporadic	Hereditary	Sporadic
Plasma				
Free Metanephrines	97	99	96	82
Catecholamines	69	92	89	72
Urine				
Metanephrines	96	97	82	45
Catecholamines	79	91	96	75
Total Metanephrines	60	88	97	89
Vanilmandelic acid	46	77	99	86

Table 3. The sensitivity and specificity values of diagnostic tests.

4.3 Patterns of biochemical test results

Patients with pheochromocytoma usually have larger relative increases in metanephrines than catecholamines, whereas patients with false-positive results due sympathoadrenal activation usually have larger increases in catecholamines than metanephrines. These differences are possible because pheochromocytoma tumor cells produce metanephrines continuously and release into the circulation independently of variations in release of the parent catecholamines (Eisenhofer et al., 1998).

A plasma normetanephrine to NE ratio above 0.52 or a metanephrine to E ratio above 4.2 can provide confirmatory evidence of pheochromocytoma in up to 30% of patients where increases in plasma metanephrines are insufficient to prove the tumor (Eisenhofer et al., 2003).

4.4 Clonidine-suppression testing

This test was introduced by Bravo *et al.* (Bravo et al., 1981) to distinguish patients with pheochromocytoma from those with false-positive biochemical results. Decreases in elevated NE concentrations after clonidine suggest sympathetic activation, whereas a lack of decrease suggests pheochromocytoma. However, normal suppression occurs and this test is recommended for patients with plasma catecholamine levels over 1000 ng/liter (5.9

nmol/liter), with a normal response defined as a fall to within normal range (Bravo & Gifford, 1984).

Another criterion for a normal response has been a fall in plasma NE after clonidine of more than 50% in patients with normal or only mildly elevated plasma NE levels (Bravo & Tagle, 2003). Plasma normetanephrine is better than NE as end-point marker for the clonidine-supression test, because pheochromocytomas cause larger, more consistent, and less episodic increases of plasma normetanephrine than NE. 76% of plasma normetanephrine is derived from NE released by sympathetic nerves while 90% of circulating metanephrine is normally derived from metabolism of E within adrenal chromaffin cells. Lack of decrease of plasma normetanephrine combined with a high plasma level after clonidine establishes high probability of pheochromocytoma. Plasma normetanephrine concentrations remained elevated after clonidine in 96% of patients with pheochromocytoma compared with only 67% for NE. (Bravo et al., 1981; Eisenhofer et al., 2003).

4.5 Imaging

Computed tomography (CT) and magnetic resonance imaging (MRI) are sensitive studies and are recommended for initial tumor localization. MRI is preferred for children, pregnant or lactating women, anyone who expresses concern about excessive radiation exposure, and individuals who have had previous surgical resection in abdominal, pelvic, and thoracic cavities. The tumor diameter in majority of pheochromocytomas is greater than 2 cm, thus it is possible diagnose them by CT. The CT sensibility for pheochromocytoma diagnosis is about 90%. However, CT is less sensitive in small tumors. The MRI has a sensibility of 95% for the adrenal tumor bigger than 0.5 cm (Timmers et al., 2009).

Functional imaging agents that target the catecholamine synthesis, storage, and secretion pathways of chromaffin tumor cells are currently used. These techniques include $^{123/131}$ metaiodobenzylguanidine (MIBG) scintigraphy, 6-[^{18}F]fluoro-L-3,4-dihydroxyphenylalanine (DOPA) positron emission tomography (PET), and 6-[^{18}F]fluorodopamine (FDA) PET. Another modality for localization of metastatic paraganglioma is the 2-[^{18}F]fluoro-2-deoxy-D-glucose (FDG) PET, that is less tissuspecific than the other functional approaches (Timmers et al., 2009).

The ^{123}I-metaiodobenzylguanidine (MIBG) scan has better specificity than CT and MRI, however it is less sensitive in the context of familial paraganglioma syndrome, paragangliomas, and metastatic disease. ^{123}I-MIBG is preferred over ^{131}I-MIBG because of its higher sensitivity, lower radiation exposure, and improved imaging quality with single-photon emission-computed tomography (Timmers et al., 2009). Previous studies suggest a sensitivity of ^{123}I-MIBG scintigraphy of 92-98% for nonmetastatic paraganglioma and 57-79% for metastases (Van Der Horst-Schrivers et al., 2006). Recently a study confirmed that the sensitivity is high for primary tumors and relatively poor (50%) for metastases (Timmers et al., 2009).

Non-metastatic paragangliomas are well localized by these techniques described previously according to Timmers and collaborators (Timmers et al., 2009). However, for the detection of metastases seen on CT, ^{18}F-FDA-PET was superior to ^{18}F-DOPA-PET and ^{123}I-MIBG scanning. ^{18}F-FDG-PET is superior in evaluating metastatic paraganglioma with mutations in succinate dehydrogenase subunit B (SDHB), whereas ^{18}F-DOPA-PET performs best in non-SDHB patients (Timmers et al., 2007). The figure 1 shows the algorithm for biochemical and radiological diagnosis of pheochromocytoma.

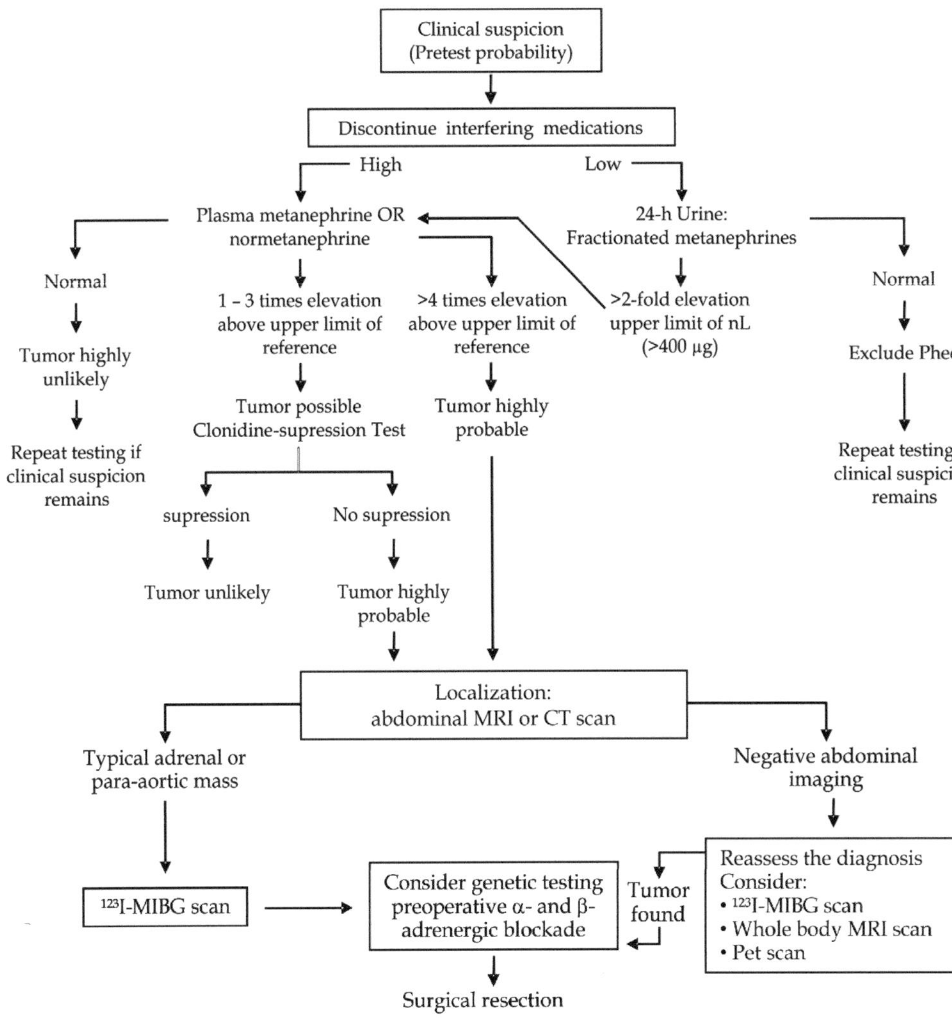

Fig. 1. The algorithm for biochemical and radiological diagnosis of pheochromocytoma.

4.6 Genetics

In actuality, 17 - 35% of pheochromocytomas and paragangliomas have a hereditary background. These hereditary tumors have been described in patients with neurofibromatosis type 1 (NF1), von Hippel Lindau syndrome (VHL), multiple endocrine neoplasia type 2 (MEN 2), and paraganglioma/ pheochromocytoma syndromes types 1-4 (PGL1, PGL2, PGL3, and PGL4) (Gill et al., 2011). The mutated genes are, respectively, NF1, VHL, RET proto-oncogene (Rearranged in Transfection), and subunits of the enzyme succinate dehydrogenase (SDHD, SDH5, SDHC, and SDHB) (Gimenez-Roqueplo et al., 2003). Hereditary pheochromocytomas and paragangliomas can be found at any age. However, most of these tumors are diagnosed in people younger than 50 years of age (Eisenhofer et al., 2011a). The most prevalent among these syndromes is PGL 1, caused by germline SDHD mutations, followed by PGL 4, whereas PGL 3 is rare (Amar et al., 2005).

The genetic screening should be considered in patients with history for paraganglial tumors, multiple tumors, young age at diagnosis, malignant pheochromocytoma because the prognosis in carriers of SDHB mutations is worse compared with non-SDHB-positive ones (Jiménez et al., 2006). Identification of a patient as a carrier of a germline mutation should be as early as possible. Mutation analysis of NF1 gene is not indicated because patients who have pheochromocytoma and carry this gene mutation also have neurofibromas or other signs of the syndrome. In general, patients presenting with pheochromocytoma who have MEN 2 and a RET mutation will have a personal or family history of MEN 2 features (Eisenhofer et al., 2011b). Mutations of VHL, NF 1 and RET genes are rare. Therefore, mutation analysis of VHL, RET, and NF 1 should not be performed unless there is clear clinical evidence of these syndromic features in the patient and/or family (Neumann & Eng, 2010).

The pathological examination of surgically resected or biopsied tumor tissue or a diagnosis of inoperable malignant pheochromocytoma based on findings of metastatic disease by imaging studies is required to confirm pheochromocytoma.

5. References

Amar, L.; Bertherat, J.; Baudin, E, Ajzenberg, C.; Bressac-de Paillerets, B.; Chabre, O.; Chamontin, B.; Delemer, B.; Giraud, S.; Murat, A.; Niccoli-Sire, P.; Richard, S.; Rohmer, V.; Sadoul, J.L.; Strompf, L.; Schlumberger, M.; Bertagna, X.; Plouin, PF.; Jeunemaitre, X. & Gimenez-Roqueplo, A.P. (2005). Genetic testing in pheochromocytoma or functional paraganglioma. *J Clin Oncol.* Vol.23, No. 34, (December 2005), pp. 8812-8. ISSN: 0732-183X.

Beard, C.M.; Sheps, S.G.; Kurland, L.; Carney, J.A. & Lie, J.T. (1983). Occurrence of pheochromocytoma in Rochester, Minnesota, 1950 through 1979. *Mayo Clin Proc.* Vol. 58, No. 12, (December 1983), pp. 802-4. ISSN: 0025-6196.

Bravo, E.L.; Tarazi, R.C.; Gifford, R.W. & Stewart, B.H. (1979). Circulating and urinary catecholamines in pheochromocytoma. Diagnostic and pathophysiologic implications. *N Engl J Med.* Vol. 301, No. 13, (September 1979), pp. 682-6. ISSN: 0028-4793.

Bravo, E.L.; Tarazi, R.C.; Fouad, F.M.; Textor, S.C.; Gifford, R.W. Jr. & Vidt, D.G. (1982). Blood pressure regulation in pheochromocytoma. *Hypertension.* Vol. 4, No. 3 Pt 2, (May-June 1982), pp. 193-9. ISSN: 0194-911X.

Bravo, E.L. & Tagle, R. (2003). Pheochromocytoma: state-of-the-art and future prospects. *Endocr Rev.* Vol. 24, No. 4, (August 2003), pp. 539-53. ISSN: 0163-769X.

Bravo, E.L., Tarazi, R.C.; Fouad, F.M.; Vidt, D.G. & Gifford, R.W. Jr. (1981). Clonidine-suppression test: a useful aid in the diagnosis of pheochromocytoma. *N Engl J Med.* Vol. 305, No. 11, (September 1981), pp. 623-6. ISSN: 0028-4793.

Bravo, E.L. & Gifford, R.W. Jr. (1984). Current concepts. Pheochromocytoma: diagnosis, localization and management. *N Engl J Med.* Vol. 311, No. 20, (November 1984), pp. 1298-303. ISSN: 0028-4793.

Cascón, A.; Pita, G.; Burnichon, N.; Landa, I.; López-Jiménez, E.; Montero-Conde, C.; Leskelä, S.; Leandro-García, L.J.; Letón, R.; Rodríguez-Antona, C.; Díaz, J.A.; López-Vidriero, E.; González-Neira, A.; Velasco, A.; Matias-Guiu, X.; Gimenez-Roqueplo, A.P. & Robledo, M. (2009). Genetics of pheochromocytoma and paraganglioma in Spanish patients. *J Clin Endocrinol Metab.* Vol. 94, No. 5, (May 2009), pp. 1701-5. ISSN: 0021-972X.

deS Senanayake, P.; Denker, J.; Bravo, E.L. & Graham, R.M. (1995). Production, characterization, and expression of neuropeptide Y by human pheochromocytoma. *J Clin Invest.* Vol. 96, No. 5, (November 1995), pp. 2503-9. ISSN: 0021-9738.

Eisenhofer, G.; Goldstein, D.S.; Walther, M.M.; Friberg, P.; Lenders, J.W.; Keiser, H.R. & Pacak, K. (2003). Biochemical diagnosis of pheochromocytoma: how to distinguish true- from false-positive test results. *J Clin Endocrinol Metab.* Vol. 88, No. 6, (June 2003), pp. 2656-66. ISSN: 0021-972X.

Eisenhofer, G.; Keiser, H.; Friberg, P.; Mezey, E.; Huynh, T.T.; Hiremagalur, B.; Ellingson, T.; Duddempudi, S.; Eijsbouts, A. & Lenders, J.W. (1998). Plasma metanephrines are markers of pheochromocytoma produced by catechol-O-methyltransferase within tumors. *J Clin Endocrinol Metab.* Vol. 83, No. 6, (June 1998), pp. 2175-85. ISSN: 0021-972X.

Eisenhofer, G.; Lenders, J.W.; Linehan, W.M.; Walther, M.M.; Goldstein, D.S. & Keiser, H.R. (1999). Plasma normetanephrine and metanephrine for detecting pheochromocytoma in von Hippel-Lindau disease and multiple endocrine neoplasia type 2. *N Engl J Med.* Vol. 340, No. 24, (June 1999), pp. 1872-9. ISSN: 0028-4793.

Eisenhofer, G.; Timmers, H.J.; Lenders, J.; Bornstein, S.R.; Tiebel, O.; Mannelli, M.; King, K.S.; Vocke, C.D.; Linehan, W.M.; Bratslavsky, G. & Pacak, K. (2011). Age at diagnosis of pheochromocytoma differs according to catecholamine phenotype and tumor location. *J Clin Endocrinol Metab.* Vol. 96, No. 2, (February 2011), pp. 375-84. ISSN: 0021-972X.

Eisenhofer, G.; Lenders, J.W.; Timmers, H.; Mannelli, M.; Grebe, S.K.; Hofbauer, L.C.; Bornstein, S.R.; Tiebel, O.; Adams, K.; Bratslavsky, G.; Linehan, W.M. & Pacak, K. (2011). Measurements of plasma methoxytyramine, normetanephrine, and metanephrine as discriminators of different hereditary forms of pheochromocytoma. *Clin Chem.* Vol. 57, No. 3, (March 2011), pp. 411-20. ISSN: 0009-9147.

Erickson, D.; Erickson D, Kudva, Y.C.; Ebersold, M.J.; Thompson, G.B.; Grant, C.S.; van Heerden, J.A. & Young, W.F. Jr. (2001). Benign paragangliomas: clinical presentation and treatment outcomes in 236 patients. *J Clin Endocrinol Metab.* Vol. 86, No. 11, (November 2001), pp. 5210-6. ISSN: 0021-972X.

Gagel, R.F.; Tashjian, A.H. Jr; Cummings, T.; Papathanasopoulos, N.; Kaplan, M.M.; DeLellis, R.A.; Wolfe, H.J. & Reichlin, S. (1988). The clinical outcome of prospective screening for multiple endocrine neoplasia type 2a. An 18-year experience. *N Engl J Med.* Vol. 318, No. 8, (February *1988)*, pp. 478-84. ISSN: 0028-4793.

Gill, A.J.; Pachter, N.S.; Clarkson, A.; Tucker, K.M.; Winship, I.M.; Benn, D.E.; Robinson, B.G. & Clifton-Bligh, R.J. (2011). Renal tumors and hereditary pheochromocytoma-paraganglioma syndrome type 4. *N Engl J Med.* Vol. 364, No. 9, (March 2011), pp. 885-6. ISSN: 0028-4793.

Gimenez-Roqueplo, A.P.; Favier, J.; Rustin, P.; Rieubland, C.; Crespin, M.; Nau, V.; Khau Van Kien, P.; Corvol, P.; Plouin, P.F.; Jeunemaitre, X. & COMETE Network. (2003). Mutations in the SDHB gene are associated with extra-adrenal and/or malignant phaeochromocytomas. *Cancer Res.* Vol. 63, No. 17, (September 2003), pp. 5615-21. ISSN: 0008-5472.

Golden, S.H.; Robinson, K.A.; Saldanha, I.; Anton, B. & Ladenson, P.W. (2009). Clinical review: Prevalence and incidence of endocrine and metabolic disorders in the United States: a comprehensive review. *J Clin Endocrinol Metab.* Vol. 94, No. 6, (June 2009), pp. 1853-78. ISSN: 0021-972X.

Guerrero, M.A.; Schreinemakers, J.M.; Vriens, M.R.; Suh, I.; Hwang, J.; Shen, W.T.; Gosnell, J.; Clark, O.H. & Duh, Q.Y. (2009). Clinical spectrum of pheochromocytoma. *J Am Coll Surg.* Vol. 209, No. 6, (December 2009), pp. 727-32. ISSN: 1072-7515.

Jiménez, C. (2010). A current review of the etiology, diagnosis, and treatment of pediatric pheochromocytoma and paraganglioma. *J Clin Endocrinol Metab.* Vol. 95, No. 5, (May 2010), pp. 2023-37. ISSN: 0021-972X.

Jiménez, C.; Cote, G.; Arnold, A. & Gagel, R.F. (2006). Review: Should patients with apparently sporadic pheochromocytomas or paragangliomas be screened for hereditary syndromes? *J Clin Endocrinol Metab.* Vol. 91, No. 8, (August 2006), pp. 2851-8. ISSN: 0021-972X.

Kopetschke, R.; Slisko, M.; Kilisli, A.; Tuschy, U.; Wallaschofski, H.; Fassnacht, M.; Ventz, M.; Beuschlein, F.; Reincke, M.; Reisch, N. & Quinkler, M. (2009). Frequent incidental discovery of phaeochromocytoma: data from a German cohort of 201 phaeochromocytoma. *Eur J Endocrinol.* Vol. 161, No. 2, (August 2009), pp. 355-61. ISSN: 0804-4643.

Kudva, Y.C.; Sawka, A.M. & Young, W.F Jr. (2003). Clinical review 164: The laboratory diagnosis of adrenal pheochromocytoma: the Mayo Clinic experience. *J Clin Endocrinol Metab.* Vol. 88, No. 10, (October 2003), pp. 4533-9. ISSN: 0021-972X.

Lenders, J.W.; Pacak, K.; Walther, M.M.; Linehan, W.M.; Mannelli, M.; Friberg, P.; Keiser, H.R.; Goldstein, D.S. & Eisenhofer, G. (2002). Biochemical diagnosis of pheochromocytoma: which test is best? *JAMA.* Vol. 287, No. 11, (March 2002), pp. 1427-34. ISSN: 0098-7484.

Lenders, J.W.; Eisenhofer, G.; Mannelli, M. & Pacak, K. (2005). Phaeochromocytoma. *Lancet.* Vol. 366, No. 9486, (August 2005), pp. 665-75. ISSN: 0140-6736.

Lundberg, J.M.; Hökfelt, T.; Hemsén. A.; Theodorsson-Norheim, E.; Pernow, J.; Hamberger, B. & Goldstein, M. (1986). Neuropeptide Y-like immunoreactivity in adrenaline cells of adrenal medulla and in tumors and plasma of pheochromocytoma patients. *Regul Pept.* Vol 13, No. 2, (January 1986), pp. 169-82. ISSN: 0167-0115.

Lundberg, J.M. & Tatemoto, K. (1982). Pancreatic polypeptide family (APP, BPP, NPY and PYY) in relation to sympathetic vasoconstriction resistant to alpha-adrenoceptor blockade. *Acta Physiol Scand.* Vol. 116, No. 4, (December 1982), pp. 393-402. ISSN: 1748-1708.

Madani, R.; Al-Hashmi, M.; Bliss, R. & Lennard, T.W. (2007). Ectopic pheochromocytoma: does the rule of tens apply? *World J Surg.* Vol. 31, No. 4, (April 2007), pp. 849-54. Erratum in: *World J Surg.* Vol. 32, No. 2, (February 2008), pp. 334. ISSN: 0364-2313.

Mannelli, M. (1989). Diagnostic problems in pheochromocytoma. *J Endocrinol Invest.* Vol. 12, No. 10, (November 1989), pp. 739-57. ISSN: 0391-4097.

Mannelli, M.; Castellano, M.; Schiavi, F.; Filetti, S.; Giacchè, M.; Mori, L.; Pignataro, V.; Bernini, G.; Giachè, V.; Bacca, A.; Biondi, B.; Corona, G.; Di Trapani, G.; Grossrubatscher, E.; Reimondo, G.; Arnaldi, G.; Giacchetti, G.; Veglio, F.; Loli, P.; Colao, A.; Ambrosio, M.R.; Terzolo, M.; Letizia, C.; Ercolino, T. & Opocher, G. Italian Pheochromocytoma/Paraganglioma Network. (2009). Clinically guided genetic screening in a large cohort of italian patients with pheochromocytomas and/or functional or nonfunctional paragangliomas. *J Clin Endocrinol Metab.* Vol. 94, No. 5, (May 2009), pp. 1541-7. ISSN: 0021-972X.

McNeil, A.R.; Blok, B.H.; Koelmeyer, T.D.; Burke, M.P.; & Hilton, J.M. (2000). Phaeochromocytomas discovered during coronial autopsies in Sydney, Melbourne and Auckland. *Aust N Z J Med.* Vol. 30, No. 6, (December 2000), pp. 648-52. ISSN: 0004-8291.

Neumann, H.P.; Bausch, B.; McWhinney SR.; Bender, B.U.; Gimm, O.; Franke, G.; Schipper, J.; Klisch, J.; Altehoefer, C.; Zerres, K.; Januszewicz, A.; Eng, C.; Smith, W.M.; Munk, R.; Manz, T.; Glaesker, S.; Apel, T.W.; Treier, M.; Reineke, M.; Walz, M.K.; Hoang-Vu, C.; Brauckhoff, M.; Klein-Franke, A.; Klose, P.; Schmidt, H.; Maier-Woelfle, M.; Peçzkowska, M.; Szmigielski, C.; Eng, C. & Freiburg-Warsaw-Columbus. Pheochromocytoma Study Group. (2002). Germ-line mutations in nonsyndromic pheochromocytoma. *N Engl J Med.* Vol. 346, No. 19, (May 2002), pp. 1459- 66. ISSN: 0028-4793.

Neumann, H.P.H. & Eng, C. (2010). Management of paraganglioma, *In: A Clinical Approach to Endocrine Metabolic Diseases.* Ladenson P.W. pp. 197-208. The Endocrine Society, ISBN: 1-879225-70-0, Chevy Chase, Maryland

O'Hare, M. & Schwartz, T.W. (1989). Expression and precursor processing of neuropeptide Y in human pheochromocytoma and neuroblastoma tumors. *Cancer Res.* Vol. 49, No. 24 Pt 1, (December 1989), pp. 7010-4. ISSN: 0008-5472.

Omura, M.; Saito, J.; Yamaguchi, K.; Kakuta, Y. & Nishikawa, T. (2004). Prospective study on the prevalence of secondary hypertension among hypertensive patients visiting a general outpatient clinic in Japan. *Hypertens Res.* Vol. 27, No. 3, (March 2004), pp. 193-202. ISSN: 0916-9636.

Perel, Y.; Schlumberger, M.; Marguerite, G.; Alos, N.; Revillon, Y.; Sommelet, D.; De Lumley, L.; Flamant, F.; Dyon, J.F.; Lutz, P.; Heloury, H. & Lemerle, J. (1997). Pheochromocytoma and paraganglioma in children: a report of 24 cases of the French Society of Pediatric Oncology. *Pediatr Hematol Oncol.* Vol. 14, No. 5, (September-October 1997), pp. 413-22. ISSN: 1077-4114.

Sawka, A.M.; Jaeschke, R.; Singh, R.J. & Young, W.F. Jr. (2003). A comparison of biochemical tests for pheochromocytoma: measurement of fractionated plasma metanephrines compared with the combination of 24-hour urinary metanephrines and catecholamines. *J Clin Endocrinol Metab.* Vol. 88, No. 2, (February 2003), pp. 553-8. ISSN: 0021-972X.

Shen, W.T.; Grogan, R.; Vriens, M.; Clark, O.H. & Duh, Q.Y. (2010). One hundred two patients with pheochromocytoma treated at a single institution since the introduction of laparoscopic adrenalectomy. *Arch Surg.* Vol. 145, No. 9, (September 2010), pp. 893-7. ISSN: 0004-0010.

Smythe, G.A.; Edwards, G.; Graham, P. & Lazarus, L. (1992). Biochemical diagnosis of pheochromocytoma by simultaneous measurement of urinary excretion of epinephrine and norepinephrine. *Clin Chem.* Vol. 38, no. 4, (April 1992), pp. 486-92. ISSN: 0009-9147.

Stenström, G & Svärdsudd, K. (1986). Pheochromocytoma in Sweden 1958-1981. (1986). An analysis of the National Cancer Registry Data. *Acta Med Scand.* Vol. 220, No. 3, (1986), pp. 225-32. ISSN: 0003-9926

Suh, I.; Shibru, D.; Eisenhofer, G.; Pacak, K.; Duh, Q.Y.; Clark, O.H. & Kebebew, E. (2009). Candidate genes associated with malignant pheochromocytomas by genome-wide expression profiling. *Ann Surg.* Vol. 250, No. 6, (December 2009), pp. 983-90. ISSN: 0003-4932.

Timmers, H.J.; Chen, C.C.; Carrasquillo, J.A.; Whatley, M.; Ling, A.; Havekes, B.; Eisenhofer, G.; Martiniova, L.; Adams, K.T. & Pacak, K. (2009) Comparison of 18F-fluoro-L-DOPA, 18F-fluoro-deoxyglucose, and 18F-fluorodopamine PET and 123I-MIBG scintigraphy in the localization of pheochromocytoma and paraganglioma. *J Clin Endocrinol Metab.* Vol. 94, No.12 (December 2009), pp. 4757-67. ISSN: 0021-972X.

Timmers, H.J.; Kozupa, A.; Chen, C.C.; Carrasquillo, J.A.; Ling, A.; Eisenhofer, G.; Adams, K.T.; Solis, D.; Lenders, J.W. & Pacak, K. (2007). Superiority of fluorodeoxyglucose positron emission tomography to other functional imaging techniques in the evaluation of metastatic SDHB-associated pheochromocytoma and paraganglioma. *J Clin Oncol.* Vol. 25, No. 16, (June 2007), pp. 2262-9. ISSN: 0732-183X.

Van Der Horst-Schrivers, A.N.; Jager, P.L.; Boezen, H.M.; Schouten, J.P.; Kema, I.P. & Links, T.P. (2006). Iodine-123 metaiodobenzylguanidine scintigraphy in localizing phaeochromocytomas--experience and meta-analysis. *Anticancer Res.* Vol. 26, No. 2B, (March-April 2006), pp. 1599-604. ISSN: 0250-7005.

Van Der Horst-Schrivers, A.N.; Osinga, T.E.; Kema, I.P.; Van Der Laan, B.F. & Dullaart, R.P. (2010). Dopamine excess in patients with head and neck paragangliomas. *Anticancer Res.* Vol. 30, No. 12, (December 2010), pp. 5153-8. ISSN: 0250-7005.

Villar, J.M.; Moreno, P.; Ortega, J.; Bollo, E.; Ramírez, C.P.; Muñoz, N.; Martínez, C.; Domínguez-Adame, E.; Sancho, J.; del Pino, J.M.; Couselo, J.M.; Carrión, A.; Candel, M.; Cáceres, N.; Octavio, J.M.; Mateo, F.; Galán, L.; Ramia, J.M.; Aguiló, J. & Herrera, F. (2010). Results of adrenal surgery. Data of a Spanish National Survey.

Langenbecks Arch Surg. Vol. 395, No. 7, (September 2010), pp. 837-43. ISSN: 1435-2443.

Young, W.F. & Sheps, S.G. (2008). Management of Pheochomocytoma, *In: Hypertension Prime. The Essentials of High Blood Pressure: Basic Science, population science, and clinical management.* Joseph L Izzo Jr, Domenic A Sica, Henry R Black (eds) pp. 571-573. Fourth Edition. Lippincott Williams & Wilkins, American Heart Association, ISBN: 978-0-7817-8205-0. Dallas, Texas.

Part 6

Treatment and Clinical Cases

10

Undiagnosed Pheochromocytoma Complicated with Perioperative Hemodynamic Crisis and Multiple Organ Failure

Anis Baraka
American University of Beirut
Beirut
Lebanon

1. Introduction

Pheochromocytoma is a rare catecholamine secreting tumor of the chromaffin of the body derived from the neural crest tissue and accounts for 0.1% to 1% of all cases of chronic hypertension (Manger et al, 1985). The common presenting signs and symptoms are paroxysmal hypertension, headache, excessive sweating, and palpitation. The hypertension is episodic in nature in up to 50% of cases. Also, 10% of patients remain normotensive (Bravo & Gifford, 1984). Thus, pheochromocytoma may go unrecognized and up to 50% of the cases are diagnosed only at postmortem examination. A proportion of patients are diagnosed at the time of incidental surgery, when induction of anesthesia and surgical manipulations may precipitate catastrophic hemodynamic crisis and even multiple organ failure (Siddik-Sayyid et al. 2007; Dabbous et al.2007; O'Riordan JA, 1997). In this situation, mortality is close to 80% (O'Riordan, 1997). The dramatic improvement in surgical outcome of diagnosed pheochromocytoma can be attributed to adequate preoperative imaging, appropriate medical preparation, and improved surgical and anesthetic techniques (Schiff & Welsh, 2003).

2. Pheochromocytoma the "10% tumor"

Pheochromocytoma has been referred to as the "10% tumor" because 10% are extraadrenal, 10% are malignant, 10% bilateral, 10% in children, and finally 10% are hereditary. The extra-adrenal tumors are more likely to be multiple and malignant.

3. Plasma catecholamines

Plasma adrenaline concentrations >400 pg/ml, and plasma noradrenaline concentrations> 1000 pg/ml are generally diagnostic of pheochromocytoma. However, there is no significant correlation between the plasma catecholamine levels and the degree of hypertension. This may be attributed to different factors such as the decreased blood volume in the pheochromocytoma patient, the episodic secretion of catecholamines, the associated down regulation of the adrenergic receptors, as well as the paroxysmal attacks of hypertension. The presence of normotension despite an increased plasma concentration of catecholamines presumably reflects a decrease in the number of alpha-adrenergic receptors (down regulation) in response to increased circulating concentration of the neurotransmitter. Clonidine (0.3mg orally, suppresses the plasma concentrations of catecholamines in a hypertensive patient but not in the pheochromocytoma patient. Clonidine acts as α2-adrenergic agonist and hence can suppress an increase in the plasma catecholamine resulting from neurogenic release, but not secondary to diffusion of excess catecholamines from a pheochromocytoma into the circulation (Bravo & Gifford, 1984)

4. Preoperative preparation

Patients with pheochromocytoma are chronically vasoconstricted as a result of the high levels of circulating catecholamines, and have a secondary decrease in their blood volume. Preparation for surgery in patients with diagnosed pheochromocytoma should begin at least 2 weeks preoperatively to allow full alpha-adrenergic blockade along with the gradual restoration of blood volume. A standard protocol for adrenergic blockade is to administer phenoxyhenzamine, starting at a dose of 40mg per day, and gradually increasing to 80-120 mg per day. This single precaution may decrease perioperative mortality down from 43% to 3%. The most common side effect of phenoxybenzamine is postural hypotension. Beta-blockade can be given after starting alpha-blockade, if tachycardia or other arrhythmias develop. Beta-blockers must never be started prior to adequate alpha-blockade, since in the absence of beta2 mediated vasodilation, profound unopposed alpha-mediated vasoconstriction may lead to hypertensive crisis or pulmonary edema (MyKlejard, 2004; Kinney et al. 2002; O'Riordan, 2007; Geogheghan et al. 1998).

Whereas norepinephrine released from sympathetic nerve fibers activates the junctional α_1-adrenergic receptors, it is thought that the α_2-receptors are extrajunctional, and are preferentially stimulated by circulating catecholamines (Hamdan & Limbird, 1996). Also the α_2-receptors are located prejunctional and function as a negative feedback. Despite its selective α_1-receptor antagonist effect, prazosin has little or no α_2-receptor blocking effect at concentrations achieved clinically (Hamdan & Limbird, 1996). Nicholson and colleagues found that pheochromocytoma patients pretreated with prazosin exhibited marked hypertensive responses to tumor handling requiring phentolamine (Nicholson et al. 1983). In another study by Russel and colleagues, phenoxybenzamine, which is a nonselective α_1 and α_2-receptor blocker, provided superior intraoperative stability compared to prazosin (Russell et al. 1998). Also, in contrast to phenoxybenzamine, prazosin has a short elimination half-life (2-3 hours); therefore prazosin blood concentrations may decrease to ineffective levels at the time of surgery (Prys-Roberts, 2000).

Prys-Roberts suggested that doxazosin, a long-acting and selective α_1-adrenergic blocking agent is preferable to phenoxybenzamine when used in the dose range 2-8 mg/day. He suggests that because doxazosin does not block α_2-adrenergic activity, many patients do not require β-adrenergic blocking agents. The selective α1-antagonsist prazosin and doxazosin have been used in the management of pheochromocytoma. They do not block the presynaptic α_2-adrenergic receptors; thus by allowing norepinephrine reuptake by nerve endings, the tachycardia following the administration of the nonselective α_1 and α_2 adrenergic blocker phenoxybenzamine does not occur. However, it has the disadvantage of being long-acting and the patient may develop postoperative hypotension refractory to norepinephrine (Nicholson et al.,1983; Hull, 1986). To help assess the adequacy of preoperative management of pheochromocytoma, the following Roizen criteria should be met in order to reduce perioperative morbidity and mortality (Table 1) (Roizen et al., 1982).

Roizen et al proposed treatment for at least 10 days and until:

1. There are no marked symptoms
2. Arterial blood pressure does not exceed 160/90 mmHg on more than four measurements in 24hr
3. Systolic blood pressure has decreased by at least 15% when moving from lying to standing position, but was more than 80/45 mmHg
4. The ECG was free of changes in ST segment and T wave for 2 weeks

---

Table 1. Preoperative Preparation

There is no accepted rule regarding the duration of adequate preoperative preparation; however, the study of Russels et al suggested that 5-7 days will be generally sufficient. MFH James practice is to increase α-blockade on a daily basis until adequate hemodynamic control is achieved and then to proceed to surgery, rather than use any predetermined time period. Failure to achieve adequate control by medical means, particularly in patients with large tumors, may be an indication for relatively urgent surgery as the only mechanism for controlling the excessive catecholamine production. Also, catecholamine-induced cardiomyopathy, as well as ST and T-wave abnormalities appear to have little advantage in attempting to control them with medical management prior to tumor excision. These changes generally regress once the catecholamine source is removed (James, 2010).
Alpha-adrenergic blockade attenuates or prevents catecholamine-induced vasoconstriction, leading to decreased blood pressure as well as to expansion of the blood volume. Satisfactory alpha blockade is implied if the hematocrit decreases by about 5%, for example from 45% to 40%. Serial monitoring of the hematocrit is a useful method of evaluating the adequacy of intravascular volume expansion. Normalization of the intravascular blood volume and blood pressure by the alpha adrenergic blockade before surgery can decrease the risk of intraoperative hypertension during manipulation of the tumor, and may even decrease the degree of hypotension following excision of the tumor. Continuation of alpha adrenergic blockade therapy until the day of surgery is recommended in order to minimize the hypertensive response during surgery. Also, because of the expanded blood volume, concern that sustained alpha blockade could contribute to refractory hypotension when vascular isolation of the tumor is accomplished has not been substantiated (Stoelting & Dierdorf, 1993).

5. Undiagnosed pheochromocytoma

The classic symptoms of pheochromocytoma consist of the triad of excessive sweating, headache and palpitation, in addition to paroxysmal hypertension. However, all three symptoms occur together in less than 50% of patients. Also, hypertension may be sustained in 50% of patients who will be managed as essential hypertension. Also, patients who present with anxiety, palpitation, sweating and tremors may be misdiagnosed as stressed or menopausal. Abdominal pain, presumably due to bowel ischemia may lead to the erroneous diagnosis of acute abdomen. Hyperglycemia may occur and the patient is diagnosed as

diabetic (James, 2010). In all these situations, the diagnosis of pheochromocytoma may be missed, and hence the patient can develop severe pheochromocytoma crisis during incidental surgery or during pregnancy.
Anesthesia and surgery in unsuspected cases have a high reported mortality. In a postmortem series, 27% of patients with undiagnosed pheochromocytoma died during or shortly after surgery (Sutton et al, 1981). Headache, palpitation, sweating and hypertension are considered to be 90% predictive of pheochromocytoma (Bravo & Gifford, 1984). In practice, such symptoms are often dismissed as psychologic or stress related, and the diagnosis may be missed until the patient presents with hypertension. Also, excess catecholamines produce hyperglycemia, which may be mistaken for insulin-deficient diabetes mellitus. Even worse, patients may suffer a whole series of major cardiovascular "events" only to suffer an unheralded intraoperative pheochromocytoma crisis (Hull & Batchelor, 2003).

6. Pheochromocytoma crisis

Although less than 0.1% patients with hypertension actually have a pheochromocytoma, nearly 50% of deaths in patients with unsuspected pheochromocytoma occur during anesthesia and surgery or during parturition (Kirkendahl et al., 1965).
The factors triggering intraoperative pheochromocytoma crisis can be attributed to excessive release of catecholamines from the undiagnosed tumor secondary to anxiety of the awake patient, or secondary to light general anesthesia during surgery (Table 2).

- Anxiety of the awake patient
- Light anesthesia during tracheal intubation and surgery
- Mechanical Factors
  - Straining
  - Scrubbing
  - Abdominal manipulations of the tumor
  - CO_2 insufflation during laparoscopy
  - Excessive uterine contractions or fetal movements
- Excessive uterine contractions or fetal movements during pregnancy

Table 2. Factors precipitating pheochromocytoma crisis.

Excessive release of catecholamines may be also drug-induced secondary to histamine release, dopamine receptor blockade, or sympathomimetic action (Table 3).
In addition, excessive release of catecholamines from the pheochromocytoma may be attributed to mechanical factors such as squeeze of the tumor during straining, positioning of the patient, by scrubbing, by intraperitoneal carbon dioxide insufflations during laparoscopy, or direct manipulation of the tumor. It should be also remembered that radiocontrast media has been also associated with pheochromocytoma crisis.
In the pregnant patient, having pheochromocytoma, excessive uterine contractions or fetal movements, as well as normal vaginal delivery or Cesarean section may precipitate the crisis; the symptoms and signs may mimic that of severe preeclampsia. However, preeclampsia is associated with hypertension and proteinuria usually after the 20th week of

gestation, while pheochromocytoma is rarely associated with proteinuria and may cause hypertension throughout pregnancy (Mudsmith et al., 2006).

Anticholinergic drugs	
e.g.	atropine
Sympathomimetic drugs	
e.g.	pancuronium
Histamine releasing drugs	
e.g.	morphine
	atracurium, mivacurium
Dopamine receptor blocker	
e.g.	droperidol (inhibits reuptake of catecholamines)
Catecholamine-sensitizing anesthetics	
e.g.	halothane
	desflurane

Table 3. Drugs precipitating pheochromocytoma crisis.

The perioperative pheochromocytoma crisis may mimic other conditions such as thyroid storm (Hirvonen et al.,2004) or malignant hyperthermia (Crowley et al.,1988; Allen & Rosenberg, 1990). However, the absence of any increase of end-tidal CO_2, the lack of rigidity, and the near limited increase in temperature may exclude the diagnosis of malignant hyperthermia. The presentation of thyroid storm usually includes fever and tachycardia, with infection commonly being a precipitating factor. Profuse sweating with a high fever out of proportion to the infection may be a due to the presence of a thyroid storm. Systolic hypertension and widened pulse pressure is also a common occurrence. Dramatic changes in heart rate and/or blood pressure should alert the anesthesiologist to consider pheochromocytoma crisis as a possible cause. However, circulatory shock and/or pulmonary oedema may be the first manifestation of undiagnosed pheochromocytoma (3).
The anesthesiologist faced with a patient developing severe hypertension which may alternate with hypotension, with developing tachycardia, sweating, heart failure, pulmonary edema and acidosis should consider the diagnosis of pheochromocytoma. Another sign which may help to confirm the diagnosis is pupillary dilation due to high levels of catecholamines (Larson & Herman, 1992). Emergency treatment will usually involve shot-acting vasodilator such as the α-adrenergic blocker phentolamine. In the case of epinephrine-secreting tumor, the severe tachycardia can be controlled by the short-acting and selective B1-adrenergic blocker esmolol.

7. Incidental surgery

Occasionally, patients undergoing incidental surgery are found to have undiagnosed pheochromocytoma. This may occur when a tumor is found by the surgeon. Also, dramatic changes in heart rate and/or blood pressure should alert the anesthesiologist to consider pheochromocytoma as a cause. This will require judicious use of short-acting vasodilator drugs such as phentolamine or sodium nitroprusside to control the hypertension. Whenever hypertension is associated with extreme tachycardia, the use of short-acting and selective β1-adrenergic blocker such as esmolol may be administered. Except when there is extreme tachycardia, the use of β -blockade in this acute situation without previous α-blockade is best avoided. Where surgery can be reasonably be aborted, that is likely to be the wise option (Hull & Batchelor, 2003).

7.1 Case report (Siddik-Sayyid et al.,2007)

A 43-year-old female patient was admitted to the hospital for right modified radical mastectomy. She had a past history of headache and palpitations with no hypertension: her preoperative blood pressure (BP) was 130/80 mmHg and her heart rate (HR) was 80 beats/min. Preoperative electrocardiogram and chest x-ray were normal. General anesthesia was induced with propofol, 2 mg/kg, fentanyl, 2 μg/kg, and cisatracurium, 0.15 mg/kg, and was maintained with isoflurane in a mixture of nitrous oxide and oxygen (2:1) by using intermittent positive-pressure ventilation. Thirty minutes after the start of surgery, the patient developed severe hypertension (BP 230/135 mmHg) and marked tachycardia (HR 160-180 beats/min). The anesthetic level was deepened by increasing the concentration of isoflurane and by additional doses of fentanyl (3 μg/kg) and midazolam (2 mg). Also, intravenous boluses of nitroglycerin (100 μg) and propranolol (1 mg) were given. The BP decreased to 100/50 mmHg and the HR to 130 beats/min. Right mastectomy and lymph node dissection were continued. Twenty minutes later, oxygen saturation as monitored by pulse oximetry dropped to 92%. Also, chest auscultation revealed diffuse crepitations over both lung fields. Arterial blood gas analysis showed hypoxemia associated with uncompensated metabolic acidosis. Esophageal temperature increased to 38.5^{o}C. Surgery lasted for 2 hours, and the patient was transferred intubated and ventilated to the intensive care unit for further management.

A chest x-ray showed widespread alveolar infiltration suggestive of pulmonary edema. Echocardiography revealed severe global hypokinesia of the left ventricle with an estimated ejection fraction of 20% to 25%. Cardiac catheterization showed normal coronaries. The patient's clinical condition deteriorated rapidly; she developed MOF including acute renal failure, hepatitis, pancreatitis, and disseminated intravascular coagulation. A computed tomography (CT) scan of the abdomen showed a 5.8cm mass in the left adrenal region, which raised suspicions of a pheochromocytoma. Spot urine vanillylmandelic acid (VMA) was 50.8 μg/mg of creatinine (normal range in this laboratory is 10.4 μg/mg of creatinine) with a creatinine of 12.6 mg/dl. A presumptive diagnosis of pheochromocytoma was made.

The patient remained on mechanical ventilation and required daily hemodialysis. She was transfused with packed cells, platelets, and fresh frozen plasma. Blood cultures grew no pathogens; however, she was started on imipenem and vancomycin. The patient had marked fluctuations of BP between 85/55 mmHg and 220/120 mmHg, which necessitated aggressive inotropic support alternating with the combination of nitroglycerin and sodium nitroprusside infusion. A pulmonary artery catheter was inserted and showed a cardiac index varying between 2.3 and 3.0 L/min/m^2 and a pulmonary artery pressure varying between 26/11 and 43/22 mmHg. During the following days, the patient's temperature normalized, and there was improvement of the pulmonary, hepatic, pancreatic, and coagulation systems. However, the blood urea nitrogen and creatinine remained markedly elevated despite daily hemodialysis for 3 to 4 hours. On the 13th day after the surgery, it was decided to proceed with an emergency excision of the pheochromocytoma.

Two days before surgery, prazosin was started at a dose of 1 mg orally 3 times a day. The antihypertensive regimen was maintained until the morning of surgery. The hemodynamic profile before anesthesia showed BP of 140/70 mmHg, heart rate of 120 beats/min, and central venous pressure of 12 mmHg. In the operating room, the patient was monitored continuously with 5-lead electrocardiogram, pulse oximetry, capnography, intraarterial blood pressure, and central venous pressure measurements. Anesthesia was induced with propofol, 1 mg/kg, midazolam, 0.03 mg/kg and cisatracurium, 0.2 mg/kg, and a remifentanil infusion was initiated at a rate of 2 μg/kg.min. Anesthesia was maintained with 2% to 5% isoflurane in a mixture of air/oxygen (3:1), remifentanil, 1 to 2 μg/kg/min, and incremental doses of cisatracurium. Blood volume was expanded carefully throughout the procedure by normal saline solution to maintain an adequate central venous pressure. Through a midline abdominal incision, the left kidney was exposed, and the patient underwent resection of her left adrenal gland. During manipulation of the tumor, the BP went up to 220/120 mmHg and required increasing concentrations of isoflurane up to 6% end-tidal) and nitroprusside (1-3 μg/kg/min). The patient also developed severe tachycardia, which was controlled by intravenous esmolol, 0.5 mg/kg, followed by an intravenous infusion at a rate of 25 μg/kg/min. Ligation of the efferent vein of the tumor resulted in an abrupt fall in BP to 50/20 mmHg, which was managed with a norepinephrine infusion and rapid infusion of normal saline solution and colloid solution (Hemaccel: Hoechst Marion Roussel, Frankfurt am Main, Germany). Postoperatively, the patient made a quick recovery, and her trachea was extubated after 48 hours. Hemodialysis support was discontinued after 4 days. Pathology of the resected tissue confirmed the presence of encapsulated pheochromocytoma with focal areas of hemorrhage.

8. Pheochromocytoma during pregnancy (Hamilton,1997; Takahashi et al.,1998; Strachan et al., 2000; Mudsmith et al., 2006)

Pheochromocytoma is a dangerous condition, particularly in pregnancy, when it is difficult to diagnose, uncommon and has often been confused with preeclampsia. Pheochromocytoma during pregnancy may mimic the usual symptoms and signs of preeclampsia, either as simple hypertension or fulminant eclampsia.

Paroxysmal attacks during pregnancy may be precipitated by postural changes, the mechanical effect of the gravid uterus in the last trimester, uterine contractions during labor and increased fetal movements. Pheochromocytoma can mimic the symptoms and signs of preeclampsia and is therefore often missed. However, hypertension associated with pheochromocytoma is seldom accompanied by oedema or proteinuria, while glycosuria is often present.

The use of intravenous labetalol or hydralazine is well established in preeclampsia, and its use in combination with magnesium sulphate has been described in patients with pheochromocytoma. The pharmacodynamic properties of magnesium sulphate (direct vasodilator, inhibition of catecholamine release from the adrenal medulla) make it useful for the management of pheochromocytoma(James, 2010). Magnesium also has powerful anti-arrhythmic action in the presence of catecholamines.

When pheochromocytoma develops in pregnancy, there is a high risk of maternal and/or fetal mortality. Even vigorous fetal movements may be associated with hypertensive crisis. For cases diagnosed during pregnancy, there is a clear choice between early intervention and conservative management until fetal viability permits elective cesarean section. Hamilton et al reported the use of prazosin and propranolol followed by surgical removal of a pheochromocytoma at 7 weeks gestation, followed by an uneventful pregnancy and

delivery at 37 weeks. Nitroglycerine was used to control hypertension during surgery in preference to sodium nitroprusside on the grounds that the latter may reduce uterine blood flow. Also, phenoxyhenzamine is avoided during early pregnancy since it may have teratogenic effect.
When the pheochromocytoma is diagnosed later at 29 weeks gestation, conservative treatment using labetalol may be continued until 35 weeks when the fetus is delivered and the tumor removed at the same operation. When the parturient commences labor with unsuspected pheochromocytoma, the hypertension may be managed by intravenous phentolamine or a combination of magnesium and hydralazine until delivery, followed by oral preparation of pheochromocytoma for delayed formal resection.

9. Multicentric pheochromocytoma (Stoelting & Dierdorf, 1993; Wahlen et al., 1992; Isselbacher et al., 1994; Baraka et al., 2002)

Pheochromocytoma is a rare disorder occurring in 0.1% of the hypertensive population. It consists of a catecholamine secreting tumor, arising from chromaffin cells, either in the adrenal medulla in 75-85% of patients or in an extraadrenal location. Extraadrenal sites include any organ that contains paraganglionic tissue, along the paravertebral sympathetic chain, extending from the base of the skull to the pelvis. Most of the extraadrenal pheochromocytomas or paragangliomas are located below the diaphragm.
Pheochromocytoma hemodynamic crisis may occur in patients with undiagnosed pheochromocytoma undergoing incidental surgery, in pregnant patients, as well as in patients with multicentric extraadrenal pheochromocytoma.
Extraadrenal sites include any organ that contains paraganglionic tissue, along the paravertebral sympathetic chain extending from the base of the skull to the pelvis. Most of the extra adrenal pheochromocytomas or paragangliomas are located below the diaphragm. Approximately 18% of pheochromocytomas are extraadrenal. The most common location is the superior aortic region between the diaphragm and the inferior renal poles, in and around the renal hilum and accounts for approximately 46% of the extra adrenal tumors. Extra adrenal tumors in the inferior paraortic area between the lower renal poles and the aortic bifurcation have constituted 24% of the cases. Most of these tumors have arisen from the organ of Zucherkandl which consists of paraganglia found in the retroperitoneal region along the aorta around the inferior mesenteric artery.
Most of extraadrenal pheochromocytoma secretes norepinephrine exclusively. If both norepinephrine and epinephrine are secreted, then the pheochromocytoma is very likely to be adrenal or Zucherkandl in origin. Serious hemodynamic fluctuations may occur during manipulations of the tumor of the organ of Zucherkandl which may be attributed to excessive catecholamine release secondary to its larger size and its more difficult resection.
The present report describes the perioperative anesthetic management and the serious hemodynamic fluctuations observed in a patient undergoing resection of recurrent retroperitoneal multicentric extraadrenal pheochromocytomas. The report also shows that variable hemodynamic responses may occur during surgical excision of multicentric pheochromocytomas, suggesting that these tumors may be quite different functionally even if they grow concomitantly in the same patient.

9.1 Case report (Baraka et al. 2002)

The patient, a 28-year-old man, underwent at 12 year of age a laparotomy for the excision of an extraadrenal infrarenal pheochromocytoma adjacent to the lower pole of the left kidney.

He had been free of symptoms until three months before presentation, when he presented with paroxysmal headache, occasional sweating, palpitations, and abdominal discomfort. He was found to have a blood pressure (BP) of 200/100 mmHg. A 24-hr-urine collection showed catecholamines 5076 μg.24 hr^{-1} (normal <25μg.24 hr^{-1}), vanillylmandylic acid of 13 mg.24 hr^{-1} (normal < 8 mg.24 hr^{-1}) and metanephrines 6009 μg.24hr^{-1} (normal < 900 μg.24 hr^{-1}). Computed tomography of the abdomen revealed two retroperitoneal masses, one adjacent to the lower pole of the right kidney and a second larger mass located at the aortic bifurcation in the region of the organ of Zuckerkandl.

The patient was prepared preoperatively for two weeks with prazosin 1 mg *po* q six hours (because of the unavailability of phenoxyenazmine in our hospital), and propranolol 10 mg *tid*. The BP stabilized at 120/90 mmHg supine and standing, with a regular heart rate (HR) of 68 beats.min^{-1}. Electrocardiogram (ECG) showed normal sinus rhythm, with non-specific T wave changes in V1-V4 leads. Hematocrit (Hct) was 43% and blood sugar level was normal.

The patient was premedicated with diazepam 5 mg *po*. In the operating room, he was monitored continuously with a 5-lead ECG, pulse oximetry, capnography, intraarterial BP measurement, and pulmonary artery (PA) catheter. Prior to induction of anesthesia, BP was 145/90 mmHg and HR was 75 beats.min. General anesthesia was induced with iv lidocaine 1 mg.kg, propofol 3 mg.kg, fentanyl 2 μg/kg and rocuronium 1 mg.kg. The patient was ventilated with 4% sevoflurane in 100% O_2 prior to proceeding with laryngoscopy and tracheal intubation. Anesthesia was then maintained with 4-8% sevoflurane in 100% O_2, and by incremental doses of fentanyl and rocuronium, as needed. Blood volume was expanded throughout the procedure by lactated Ringer's solution and by Haemaccel ® (Hoechst Marion Rousse. Frankfurt am Main, Germany) to maintain adequate central venous pressure and urine output.

Through a midline abdominal incision, the right kidney was exposed and a mass was visualized, medial to the lower pole of the kidney, inferior to the renal helium and lateral to the vena cava. Dissection of the tumor from its surrounding structures was performed easily. Minimal hemodynamic changes occurred and responded to increasing concentrations of sevoflurane.

The tumor of Zuckerkandl was overlying and adherent to the bifurcation of the aorta. Surgical dissection of the tumor was difficult and associated with excessive blood loss. Manipulation of the tumor resulted in severe hypertensive episodes with BP ranging from 200/100 to 320/120 mmHg. Systemic hypertension was associated with elevation of PA pressure. Surgery was interrupted temporarily; sodium nitroprusside was infused in increasing doses up to 2μg.kg^{-1}.min^{-1}, and two doses of *iv* phentolamine 5 mg were administered. Hypertension also necessitated the bolus administration of esmolol 0.5 mg.kg^{-1} *iv* to be followed by an iv infusion of 30 mg esmolol over 20 min.

Ligation of the efferent vein of the tumor immediately resulted in a fall in BP which reached 70/50 mmHg. This hypotension was treated by decreasing the concentration of sevoflurane, as well as by rapid *iv* infusion of lactated Ringer's solution and 2 U of blood. In addition, a norepinephrine infusion (0.05 μg.kg.min) was required for 20 min. Thereafter, BP returned to normal without further treatment. The patient was kept sedated, intubated and transferred to the intensive care unit with a BP of 130/75 mmHg and a HR of 85 beats.min. His postoperative course was smooth and uneventful.

Pathology examination of the resected tumors confirmed the diagnosis of pheochromocytoma; the first mass was slightly smaller (5 x 4 x 4 cm *vs* 6 x 4 x 3.5 cm) and weighed less (43 g *vs* 46 g) than the second tumor. The two tumors showed no evidence of necrosis or unusual meiotic activity.

10. Pheochromocytoma cardiomyopathy and multiple organ failure

A high mortality rate has been reported in pheochromocytoma patients with catecholamine-induced cardiomyopathy presenting symptoms of congestive heart failure, arrhythmia, acute pulmonary oedema and nonspecific EKG changes, as well as in pheochromocytoma complicated with multiple organ failure.

Echocardiography may reveal global cardiac hypokinesia secondary to cardiomyopathy in 25% to 50% of pheochromocytoma as a result of sustained exposure of the myocardium to high levels of catecholamines. Studies have shown a global reduction in myocardial pump function caused by a down-regulated β-adrenergic receptors and a net reduction in viable myofibrils. Rabits' hearts with catecholamine-induced cardiomyopathy have shown a reduced inotropic sensitivity to noradrenaline, and also a reduced response to calcium chloride. The pathogenesis of catecholamine-induced cardiomyopathy is probably multifactorial. Catecholamine-induced vasospasm leading to hypoxia is implicated. Excess noradrenaline also induces changes in permeability of the sarcolimmal membrane leading to increased calcium influx. Also, it has been proposed that the injury process might involve release of free radicals (Sardesai et al.,1990; Gilsanz et al.., 1983; Takaror et al., 1987; Fripp et al., 1981). Left atrial enlargement secondary to catecholamine-induced left ventricular diastolic dysfunction is quite common (around 20%), but seldom poses a management problem unless accompanied by left ventricular systolic dysfunction. Left ventricular hypertrophy is frequently seen, as are ST and T-wave abnormalities. These appear to be little advantage in attempting to correct these changes by medical management prior to tumor excision. These changes generally regress once the excess catecholamines source is removed. Left ventricular failure and pulmonary edema may be present, particularly if the patient has developed signs of catecholamine-induced cardiomyopathy (James, 2010).

Multiple organ failure (MOF) may be the initial presentation, and is called pheochromocytoma multisystem crisis. MOF may result from the high levels of circulating catecholamines, which can trigger excessive vascular spasm, volume contraction, platelet aggregation and thrombosis. The splanchnic vessels are highly susceptible to catecholamine-induced vasoconstriction, and hence the ischemic gut mucosa may allow bacterial translocation or the passage of endotoxins across the intestinal barrier to extraintestinal sites including the lung which is the first organ to fail. Also, acute renal failure can be attributed to acute tubular necrosis because of the combination of cardiogenic shock reducing the renal perfusion, associated with renal vasoconstriction induced by a surge of catecholamines (Sardesai et al.,1990; Gilsanz et al.., 1983; Takaror et al., 1987; Fripp et al., 1981).

Gut-derived factors, contained primarily in the mesenteric lymph rather than the portal system, potentiate the development of distant multiple organ failure. Because the lung is the first organ exposed to mesenteric lymph, via the thoracic duct and the subclavian vein, the lung is generally the first organ to fail in severely injured patients. The role of the gut injury and loss of gut barrier function contributes to the development of a systemic inflammatory state and distant organ injury (Fukushima et al.,1998).

During the decade from 1985 to 1995, gut barrier and the ensuing translocation of bacteria and endotoxins gained acceptance as a major contribution to the development of multiple organ dysfunction syndrome (MODS). It now appears that pheochromocytoma similar to shock, trauma, or sepsis-induced gut injury can result in the gut becoming a cytokine-generating organ, and that the mesenteric circulation can become a priming bed for circulating neutrophils. Many of the same insults that cause intestinal mucosal injury and promote bacterial translocation also appear able to induce the gut and the gut-associated lymphatic tissue to produce cytokines and other inflammatory mediators that may contribute to MODS (Fukushima et al., 1998; Deitch,2001).

In a review of 54 autopsy-proven cases of unsuspected pheochromocytoma seen at the Mayo Clinic over a 50-year period, hypertensive or hypotensive crisis precipitated by surgery for unrelated conditions was a common cause of death. Intraoperative deaths have been ascribed variously to ventricular arrhythmias, wide fluctuations in systemic blood pressure, myocardial infarction, acute pulmonary oedema, and subarachnoid hemorrhage (St. John Sutton, et al.,1981). Barale et al., 1978 described two patients with circulatory shock, vasoconstriction, and pulmonary edema as the first manifestation of undiagnosed pheochromocytoma (Barale et al.,1978). Also, MOF may be the initial presentation of undiagnosed pheochromocytoma and has a poor prognosis (Barale et al.,1978; Kohle et al.,2001). Newell et al.,1988 reported 3 patients with unusual presentations of pheochromocytomas, which they called "pheochromocytoma multisystem crisis", a tetrad of symptoms including MOF, encephalopathy, high fever, and severe derangements in BP consisting of hypertension and/or hypotension. Siddik-Sayyid et al.,2007 reported a patient with an undiagnosed pheochromocytoma undergoing radical mastectomy; the patient developed intraoperative severe hemodynamic changes and pulmonary oedema, complicated by postoperative MOF; the postoperative hemodynamic instability and the persistent renal failure rapidly recovered after excision of the pheochromocytoma (Siddik-Sayyid et al., 2007).

Management of intraoperative pheochromocytoma crisis in patients undergoing incidental surgery consists of elimination of the triggering factors, as well as controlling hypertension by the administration of short-acting vasodilators such as the alpha-adrengergic blocker phentolamine, or sodium nitroprusside infusion. Whenever hypertension is associated with severe tachycardia, beta-adrenergic blocker can be administered; the short-acting and selective beta 1 blocker esmolol is preferred to the long-acting and nonselective propranolol. The administration of beta-adrenergic blocker without prior α-adrenergic blockade may be complicated by cardiac failure and pulmonary oedema secondary to its negative inotropic effect on the heart, associated with an increased after load. Initiation of nonselective beta blocker therapy without preceding alpha blockade in a patient with pheochromocytoma my precipitate a crisis with hemodynamic collapse. Nonselective beta blockade leads to loss of beta 2 receptor-mediated vasodilation, while the unopposed effects of alpha receptors causes vasoconstriction, resulting in increased after load, causing myocardial dysfunction and pulmonary oedema (Siddik-Sayyid et al., 2007). Thus, nonselective beta blockers should be avoided in any patient who could conceivably have a pheochromocytoma, until that possibility has been excluded. Also, unexplained cardiopulmonary dysfunction, and pulmonary oedema after the institution of beta blockade, should alert the anesthesiologist to the possibility of a pheochromocytoma (Sibal et al., 2006).

In patients with undiagnosed pheochromocytoma undergoing incidental surgery, many authors recommend urgent operation whenever their condition deteriorates despite maximal medical therapy. Newell et al.,1988 recommend urgent adrenalectomy when multisystem injury is present and in cases of progressive deterioration despite medical therapy. Also, Wood (Case 6-1986) stated that preparation for operation involves a balance between severity of the illness and quality of α-blockade, and suggested that certain patients undergo surgical tumor excision with incomplete α--blockade. Freier et al.,1980 recommended urgent tumor excision after brief attempts at medical stabilization in patients presenting with alternating hypertension or hypotension, severe tachycardia, cardiac arrhythmias, encephalopathy, and renal failure.

11. Conclusion

In conclusion, patients with undiagnosed pheochromocytoma undergoing incidental surgery may develop intraoperative hemodynamic crisis complicated by postoperative multiple organ failure.

Management of intraoperative pheochromocytoma crisis consists of elimination of the triggering factors, as well as the administration of short-acting vasodilators such as the alpha-adrenergic blocker phentolamine, or sodium nitroprusside infusion. The administration of beta adrenergic blocker without prior α-adrenergic blockade may be complicated by cardiac failure and pulmonary edema secondary to its negative inotropic effect associated with an increased after load.

When the pheochromocytoma is surgically accessible during incidental surgery as laparotomy, the surgeon may be tempted to excise the tumor. However, tumor handling in unprepared patients may result in dramatic increases in arterial blood pressure followed by intractable hypotension after tumor excision. A safer option is planned resection of the pheochromocytoma after confirmation of the diagnosis and optimal preoperative pharmacologic preparation. However, urgent adrenalectomy is recommended whenever multisystem injury deteriorates despite maximal medical therapy.

12. References

Allen, GC. & Rosenberg, H. (1990). Phaechromocytoma presenting as acute malignant hyperthermia - a diagnostic challenge. *Canadian Journal of Anaesthesia* 37, pp.593-5

Baraka,A.; Siddik-Sayyid, S., Jalbout, M. & Yacoub, S. (2002). Variable hemodynamic fluctuations During resection of multicenteric extraadrenal pheochromocytoma. *Canadian Journal of Anesthesia* 49, No. 7, pp. 682-686

Barale, F.; Boillot, A., Neidhart, A., et al. (1978). Pheochromocytoma et reanimation d' urgence. *Anesthesia Analgesia Reanimation* 35, pp. 233-240

Bravo, EL. & Gifford, RW. (1984). Current concepts. Pheochromocytoma: diagnosis, localization and management. *N Engl J Med* 311, pp. 1298-1303

Case 6-1986, Case records of the Massachusetts General Hospital.(1986). Weekly clinicopatholgical exercises. *N Engl J Med* 314, pp. 431-439

Crowley, KJ.; Cunningham, AJ., Canroy, B. et al. (1988). Pheochromocytoma - A presentation mimicking malignan hyperthermia. Anaesthesia 43, pp. 1031-1032

Dabbous, A.; Siddik-Sayyid, S. & Baraka, A. (2007). Catastrophic hemodynamic changes in a patient with undiagnosed pheochromocytoma undergoing abdominal hysterectomy. *Anesthesia and Analagesia* 104, pp.223-224

Deitch, EA. (2001). Role of the gut lymphatic system in multiple organ failure. Curr Opin Crit Care 7, pp. 92-98, *Lippincott Williams & Wilkins, Inc.*

Freier, DT.; Eckhauser,FE. & Harrison, TS. (1980). Pheochromocytoma: A persistently problematic and still potentially lethal disease. *Arch Surg* 115, pp. 388-391

Fripp, RR.; Lee, JC. & Downing, SE. (1981). Inotropic responsiveness of the heart in catecholamine cardiomyopathy . Am Heart J 101, pp. 17-21

Fukushima, R.; Kabayashi, S. & Okinaga, K. (1998). Bacterial translocation in multiple organ failure. *Nippon Geka Gakkai Zasshi* 99, pp. 497-503

Gilsanz, FJ.; Luengo, C., Conejero, P. et al. (1983). Cardiomyopathy and pheochromocytoma. *Anaesthesia* 38, pp. 888-891

Geoghegan, JG.; Emberton ,M., Bloom, SR. & Lynn, JA. (1998). Changing trends in the management of pheochromocytoma. *Br J Surgery* 85, pp.117-120

Hamdan, JG. & Limbird, LE. (1996). *Goodman and Gilman's.* The Pharmacological Basis of Therapeutics, 9th ed. New York. McGraw-Hill Publishers, pp. 227-229

Hamilton, A.; Sirrs,S. , Schmidt, N. & Onrot, J. (1997). Anaesthesia for phaechromocytoma in pregnancy. *Canadian Journal of Anaesthesia* 44, pp. 654-657

Hirvonen, EA.; Niskanen, LK. & Niskanen, MM. (2004). Thyroid storm prior to induction of anaesthesia. *Anaesthesia* 59, pp.1020-1022

Hull, CJ. (1986). Phaechromocytoma-diagnosis, preoperative preparation and anaesthetic management. *British Journal of Anaesthesia* 58, pp. 1453-1468

Hull, CJ. & Batchelor, AM. (2003). Anesthetic management of patient with endocrine disease. *In Wylie and Churchill Davidson's.* A Practice of Anesthesia, 7th edition, Edited by Healy TEJ, Knight PR, pp. 811-827

Isselbacher, KJ.; Braunwald, E. , Wilson, JD. et al. (1994). *Harrison's principles of Internal Medicine* 14th ed Mc Graw Hill, pp. 1926-1929

James, MFM. (2010). Adrenal Medulla. The anesthetic management of pheochromocytoma. *In Anaesthesia for patients with endocrine disease.* Edited by MFM James. Oxford University Press Chapter 8, pp. 149-168

Kinney, MA.; Narr, BJ. & Warner, MA. (2002). Perioperative management of pheochromocytoma. *Journal Cardiothoracic & Vascular Anesthesia* 16, pp. 359-369

Kirkendahl, WH., Leighty, BRD. & Culp, DA. (1965). Diagnosis and treatment of patients with pheochromocytoma. *Arch Intern Med* 115, pp. 529-36

Kolhe, N., Stores ,J., Richardson, D., et al. (2001). Hypertension due to pheochromocytoma - An unusual cause of multiorgan failure. *Nephrol Dial Transplant* 16, pp.2100-2104

Larson, MD. & Herman ,WC. (1992). Bilateral dilated nonreactive pupils during surgery in a patient with undiagnosed pheochromocytoma. *Anesthesiology* 77, pp. 200-202

Manger, WM., Gifford, RW. Jr. & Hoffmann, BB. (1985). Pheochromocytoma: A clinical and experimental overview. *Curr Probl Cancer* 9, pp. 1-89

MyKlejard, DS. (2004). Undiagnosed pheochromocytoma. The Anesthesiologist Nightmare. *Clinical Medicine & Research* Volume 2, number 1, pp. 59-62

Mudsmith, JG.; Thomas, CE. & Browne, PA. (2006). Undiagnosed pheochromocytoma mimicking severe preeclampsia in a pregnant woman at term. *International Journal of Obstetric Anesthesia* 15, pp. 240-245

Newell, KA. , Porinz,RA., Pickleman, J., et al. (1988). Pheochromocytoma - multisystem crisis - A surgical emergency. *Arch Surg* 123, pp. 956-959

Nicholson, JP. Jr., Vaughn,ED., Pickering, TG., et al. (1983). Pheochromocytoma and prazasin. *Ann Int Med* 99, pp. 477-479

O.Riordan, JA. (1997). Pheochromocytoma and anesthesia. *Int Anesthesiol Clin* 35, pp. 99-127

Prys-Roberts, C. (2000). Pheochromocytoma-recent progress in its management. *British Journal of Anaesthesia* 85, pp. 44-57

Roizen, MF., Horrigan, RW., Koike, M., Eger, El. 2nd et al. (1982). Prospective trial of four anesthetic techniques for resection of pheochromocytoma. *Anesthesiology* 57, pp. A 43

Russell, WJ., Metcalfe, JR., Tankin, AL. & Frewin, DB. (1998). The preoperative management of pheochromocytoma. *Anesth Intensive Care* 26, pp.196-200

Sardesai , SH., Mourant, AJ., Sivathandon, Y. et al. (1990). Phaechromocytoma and catecholamine induced cardiomyopathy presenting as heart failure. *Br Heart J* 63, pp. 234-237

Schiff, RL. & Welsh, GA. (2003). Perioperative evaluation and management of the patient with endocrine dysfunction. *Med Clin N* Am 87, pp. 175-92

Sibal, L., Jovanovic, A., Agarwalt , SC., Peaston, RT., et al. (2006). Pheochromocytomas presenting as acute crisis after beta blockade therapy. *Clinical Endocrinology* 65, pp.186-190

Siddik-Sayyid, SM., Dabbous, AS., Shaaban,JA., Daaboul ,DG., & Baraka, AS. (2007). Catastrophic cardiac hypokinesia and multiple-organ failure after surgery in a patient with undiagnosed pheochromocytoma: Emergency excision of the tumor. *Journal of Cardiothoracic and Vascular Anesthesia* 21 (6), pp. 863-866

St. John Sutton, MG.; Sheps, SG. & Lie, JT. (1981). Prevalence of clinically unsuspected pheochromocytoma. Review of a 50-year autopsy series. *Mayo Clin Proc* 56, pp. 354-360

Stoelting, RK. & Dierdorf, SF. (1993). *Anesthesia and Co-Existing Disease*, 3rd ed New York, Churchill Livingstone pp. 363-367

Strachan, AN.; Claydon, P. & Caunt, JA. (2000). Phaechromocytoma diagnosed during labour. *British Journal of Anaesthesia* 85, pp. 635-637

Sutton,MG., Sheps, SG. & Lie, JT. (1981). Prevalence of clinically unsuspected phaeochromocytoma. Review of a 50 year autopsy series. Mayo Clinic Procedures 56, pp. 354-360

Takahashi ,K.; Sai, Y. & Nasaka, S. (1998). Anaesthetic management for Caesarean section combined with removal of pheochromocytoma. *Eur J Anaesthesiol* 15, pp. 364-366

Takaror, C.; Tanimuro, A. & Saito, Y. (1987). Catecholamine-induced cardiomyopathy accompanied with pheochromocytoma. *Acta Pathol Jpn* 37, pp. 123-132

Wahlen, RK.; Althausen, AF. & Daniels, GH. (1992). Extraadrenal pheochromocytoma. *J Urol* 147, pp. 1-10

11

Familial Catecholamine-Secreting Tumors - Three Distinct Families with Hereditary Pheochromocytoma

Shirin Hasani-Ranjbar, Azadeh Ebrahim-Habibi and Bagher Larijani
Endocrinology and Metabolism Research Institute, Shariati Hospital, Tehran University of Medical Sciences, Tehran, Iran

1. Introduction

Phaeochromocytomas (PHEOs) and paragangliomas (PGLs) are catecholamine-secreting tumors, that arise from chromaffin cells of the adrenal medulla and extra-adrenal sites. Extra-adrenal phaeochromocytomas are called paragangliomas (Landers et al., 2005). The Prevalence of these tumors is 1:4500 and 1:1700 and an annual incidence of 3-8 cases per 1 million per year in the general population. PHEOs/PGLs arise from three anatomically parts of the neural crest derived sympathy-adrenal system: adrenal medulla, sympathetic, and parasympathetic paraganglia (Kantorovich et al., 2010). Extra-adrenal parasympathetic paragangliomas which are located predominantly in the head and neck are approximately 95% nonsecretory. Pheochromocytomas typically occur in about 85% of cases from adrenal medullary chromaffin tissue and in about 15% of cases from extra-adrenal chromaffin tissues (Elder et al., 2005).

1.1 Malignant pheochromocytoma

Malignant forms of catecholamine-secreting tumors are rare. The malignancy rate is variable, from 2.4-26%. There are no histological proofs of malignancy for such tumors to date and the only accepted criterion is the presence of metastasis. The distant metastases are usually of hematologic origin, mostly involving bone, liver and lung (Hasani-Ranjbar, 2009, 2010). The prevalence of metastasis is up to 36-50% for extra adrenal abdominal pheochromocytoma and 10% and 5% for adrenal and familial forms respectively (Whalen et al., 1992; O Riordan et al., 1996). Some studies have suggested that the presence of necrosis, vascular invasion, extensive local invasion, and high rate of mitotic figures may indicate a malignant behavior in pheochromocytoma. A recent study by Thompson used clinical features, histologic findings, and immunophenotypic studies for identifying parameters that may help distinguish benign from malignant pheochromocytoma. This is an Adrenal Gland scale Score (PASS) which is weighted for 12 specific histologic features that are more frequently identified in malignant pheochromocytoma. Tumors with PASS more than 4 were biologically more aggressive than tumors with a PASS less than 4. Some immunohistochemical markers such as Ki-67, P52, Bcl-2 were studied to differentiate malignant from benign pheochromocytoma too (Strong et al.,2008). But practically the diagnosis of malignant pheochromocytoma can only be determined by presence of recurrence or metastatic disease at a site where chromaffin cells do not normally exist.

1.2 Familial pheochromocytoma

Most pheochromocytomas represent sporadic tumors. However some patients have disease as part of a familial disorder (15-30%). Sporadic pheochromocytomas are usually unicentric and unilateral while familial pheochromocytomas are often multicentric and bilateral. Hereditary pheochromocytoma typically present at a younger age than sporadic forms (Nourmann et al 2002; Manger & Gifford, 2002).

There are several familial disorders associated with pheochromocytoma, these syndromes include von Hippel-Lindau (VHL) syndrome, multiple endocrine neoplasia type 2 (MEN2), neurofibromatosis type 1 and SDH mutation-related tumours. The approximate frequency of pheochromocytoma in these disorders is 50 percent in MEN2, 10 to 20 percent in VHL syndrome, and 0.1 to 5.7 percent with neurofibromatosis type 1 (Hasani-Ranjbar etal., 2009, Walter et al., 1999b; Dluhy, 2002). All of these syndromes have autosomal dominant inheritance (Table 1).

Multiple endocrine neoplasia type 1 (MEN1) is an autosomal dominant predisposition to tumors of the parathyroid glands, anterior pituitary, and pancreatic islet cells. pheochromocytoma is very rare in MEN1 syndrome (Brandi, 2001).

1.2.1 Multiple Endocrine Neoplasia Type 2 (MEN 2A and MEN 2B)

The prevalence of MEN2 syndrome is 2.5 per 100,000 in the general population. MEN2 is sub classified into three syndromes: MEN2A; MEN2B; and familial medullary thyroid cancer (FMTC).

Multiple endocrine neoplasia type 2 (MEN2A) is characterized by pheochromocytoma (usually bilateral and may be asynchronous), medullary thyroid carcinoma (MTC), and hyperparathyroidism due to primary parathyroid hyperplasia (Noumann et al., 1993). The respective frequency of these tumors in MEN2 is over 90 percent for medullary thyroid cancer, approximately 40 to 50 percent for pheochromocytoma, and 10 to 20 percent for multigland.

MEN2A is a heritable predisposition to medullary thyroid cancer, pheochromocytoma, and primary parathyroid hyperplasia. MEN2B shares the inherited predisposition to medullary thyroid cancer and pheochromocytoma that occurs in MEN2A. But in patients with MEN2B other clinical disorders including mucosal neuromas, typically involving the lips and tongue, and intestinal ganglioneuromas have to be considered. FMTC is a variant of MEN2A, which is associated with medullary thyroid cancer but not the other clinical manifestations of MEN2 syndromes (Brandi etal., 2001; Pacak et al., 2005). In patients with MEN2B, Medullary thyroid cancer is often more aggressive and of earlier onset than in MEN2A; so; early diagnosis and prevention are particularly critical (Donovan et al., 1989; Mathew et al., 1987).

In contrast to MEN1, early diagnosis via screening of "at-risk" family members in MEN2A kindreds is essential because medullary thyroid cancer is a life-threatening disease that can be prevented by early thyroidectomy

DNA testing has been the best screening test for this disorder since it was recognized that affected patients have germ-line mutations in the RET proto-oncogene on chromosome 10.

	MEN2	VHL	NF1	PGL	CARNEY-triad
Major Features	MTC, PCC , Primary para-thyroid hyper-plasia	PCC, PGL, Retinal angiomas, Ccerebellar hemangioblastoma, Epididymal cystadenoma, Renal and pancreatic cysts, neuroendocrine tumors, Renal cell carcinoma	café-au-lait macules,neuro-fibroma, Freckling, optic glioma. Lisch nodules (iris hamartomas), sphenoid dysplasia,	Head and neck,media-stinal, abdominal and pelvic PGL,	PGL,Gastric leiomyo-sarcoma, Pulmonary condromas
% PCC	50%	10-20%	*Rare(0.1-5.7%*	-	-
Bilateral	50-80%	50%	16%	-	-
Benign	Almost Always	95%	Most cases	SDHB is more malignant	-
Extra-adrenal PGL	Rare	Rare	Can Occur	Usual manifestation	-
Inheritance	AD	AD	AD	SDHB & SDHC & SDH%(AD), SDHD(MI)	Unknown
Gene locus	10q11.2	3p25-26	17q11.2	SDHB1p35-36 SDHC 1q23 SDHD11q23	Unknown
catecholamine phenotype	E	NE	E	NE	Unknown

Abbreviations: VHL= von Hippel Lindau, MEN= multiple endocrine neoplasia, NF=Neurofibromatosis, PGL=Paraganglioma, PCC= Pheochromocytoma; MTC: Medullary thyroid cancer, SDH=succinate dehydrogenase type B,C,or D, AD=Autosomal Dominant, NE, norepinephrine; E, epinephrine,MT=Maternal Imprinting

Table 1. Genetic conditions associated with pheochromocytoma- Clinical, biochemical and genetic facts.

Numerous activating mutations throughout the RET proto-oncogene have been documented in persons with MEN 2A and pheochromocytoma is associated most frequently with mutations in codon 634 (in exon 11). MEN 2B is associated with mutations primarily in codon 918 (in exon 16) of the RET proto-oncogene (Mulligan et al., 1994; Carlson et al.,1994).

1.2.2 VHL syndrome

Von Hippel-Lindau (VHL) disease represents an alteration on VHL protein. The major physiological function of the VHL protein is to promote degradation of hypoxia-inducible factor (HIF1) that is a major factor involved in the regulation of hypoxia-related gene transcription (Figure 1).

Von Hippel-Lindau (VHL) disease is manifested by a variety of benign and malignant tumors. The VHL phenotype includes pheochromocytoma (frequently bilateral), paraganglioma (rarely), retinal angiomas, cerebellar hemangioblastoma, epididymal cystadenoma, renal

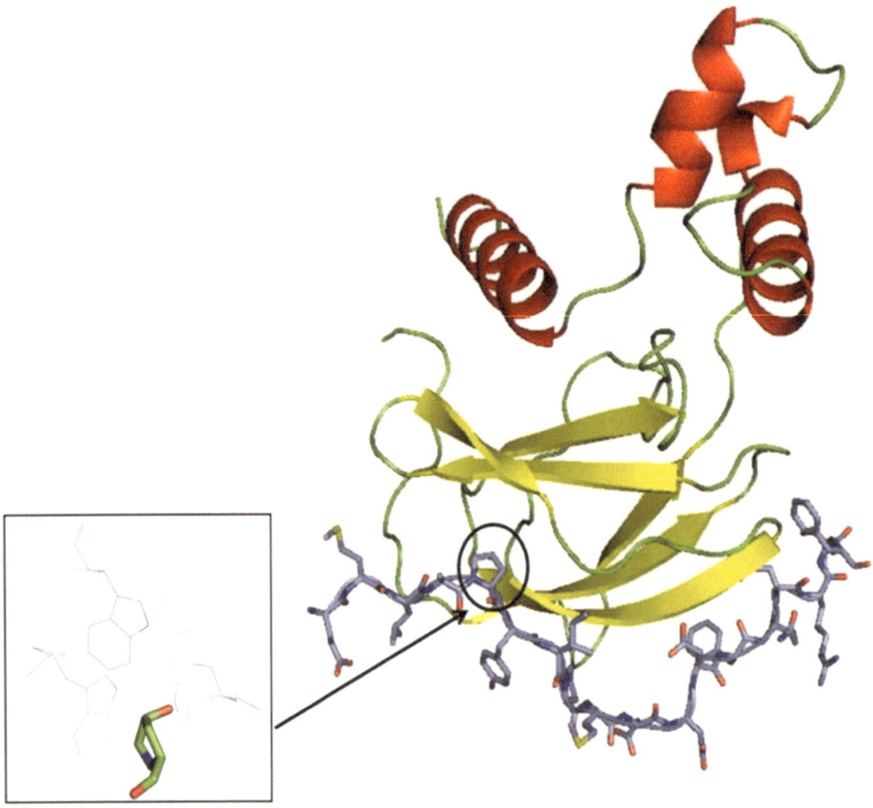

Fig. 1. pVHL (1LQB.PDB) is shown in cartoon representation, in the upper part of the picture, interacting with HIF (which residues are shown as sticks). The 564 hydroxyproline residue of HIF, which is believed to be important in the interactions between the two proteins [*REF: Science 296, 1886 (2002);Jung-Hyun Min, et al. Structure of an HIF-1a-pVHL Complex: Hydroxyproline Recognition in Signaling*] is indicated with a circle, and a view of the same hydroxyproline residue (stick) is shown in the inset image, alongside with some of the pVHL residues (labelled) that are located in its proximity. Mutations happening in these residues could be deleterious to the interaction between pVHL and HIF, and possibly involved in the disease phenotype. (This image has been created using PyMOL).

and pancreatic cysts, pancreatic neuroendocrine tumors, and renal cell carcinoma (RCC) (Hasani Ranjbar etal., 2009; Lonser et al.,2003; Patocs et al.,2008) .

VHL disease is divided into types I and II, based upon the likelihood of developing pheochromocytoma (Zbar et al., 1996). Type II families are more likely to carry a missense mutation in the VHL gene and are at higher risk for developing pheochromocytoma. Type II disease is subdivided based upon the risk of developing of RCC. Type IIA and IIB families have a low and high incidence of RCC, respectively, while type IIC kindreds are characterized by the development of pheochromocytomas only, without RCC or hemangioblastoma. Patients in kindreds with type I disease have a substantially lower risk of developing pheochromocytomas (Gomy et al., 2010).

Clinical classification of VHL include: A. Classic VHL disease (A1: Families meeting current VHL diagnostic criteria with involvement of at least three VHL tumors in two distinct organs; A2: Sporadic patients with involvement of at least two distinct tumors); B. nonclassic VHL disease, meeting criteria (B1:Families with less than 3 tumors in 2 distinct organs; B2: Cases meeting current diagnostic VHL criteria with limited VHL manifestations; C. Non classic, not meeting criteria(VHL-associated manifestations not meeting current diagnostic criteria) (Ciotti et al., 2009).

The VHL tumor suppressor gene is located on chromosome 3p25-26. More than 300 germline VHL mutations have been identified that lead to loss of function of the VHL protein (Kim & Kaelin,2004; Cruz et al., 2007). Missense, nonsense and splice site mutations, microdeletions and microinsertions are detected in approximately two-thirds of the families. Exon or entire gene deletions are found in 20-30% of the VHL families. Recently, real time quantitative PCR (RQ-PCR) and multiplex ligation-dependent probe amplification assay (MLPA) strategies have been proposed for detection of VHL deletions(Ciotti et al., 2009).

Specific VHL gene mutations appear to correlate with clinical phenotype. About 95% of patients with VHL truncating or null mutations have VHL1 (without pheochromocytoma). In patients with VHL syndrome and pheochromocytoma(VHL2) 92-98% have missense mutations.

1.2.3 Neurofibromatosis type 1

Neurofibromatosis, or NF, is the term given to two neurocutaneous genetic conditions. Neurofibromatosis type 1, also known as von Recklinghausen's is the most common type of neurofibromatosis. The incidence of approximately 1 in 2600 to 1 in 3000 individuals (Lammert et al.,2005). Approximately one-half of the cases are familial; the remainder are new mutations (North K, 1993). The hallmarks of NF1 are the multiple café-au-lait spots (CALS) and associated cutaneous neurofibromas. Pheochromocytoma has been clinically identified in 0.1 to 5.7 percent of patients with NF. The NF1 gene has been mapped to chromosome 17q11.2 and cloned (ledbetter et al 1989; Shen et al., 1996; Feldkamp et al., 1998).

Mutations in the NF1 gene result in loss of functional protein, causing the wide spectrum of clinical findings including NF1-associated tumors.

No obvious genotype-phenotype correlation between small mutations (<20 base pairs) of the NF1 gene and a specific phenotype have been demonstrated, with the exception of the c.2970-2972 delAAT (p.M990del) mutation that is associated with a very mild phenotype in the majority of cases (Upadhyaya, et al., 2007).

Genetic testing for NF1 is available but is not routinely performed, as the diagnosis is made based upon clinical phenotype.

1.2.4 Familial paraganglioma

Initial suggestion of genetic clustering of paraganglioma tumors date back to 1930, but mode of inheritance which is to be autosomal dominant with maternal imprinting in some cases was found by Van Der Mey in 1989. Later, several familial clusters of pheochromocytoma/paraganglima were described and defined as paraganglioma syndrome PGL1 through PGL4. PGL1 is to be related to mutation in the SDHD gene, PGL2 to SDH5, PGL3 to mutation in SDHC and PGL4 to SDHB. SDH-related tumorigenesis is believed to associate with hypoxia-inducible factor (HIF)/angiogenesis pathway (Kantorovich et al., 2010; López-Jiménez et al.,2010).

In this chapter three families with different forms of familial pheochromocytoma has been shown. All of the presented patients have had malignant pheochromocytoma and an unusual presentation.

2. Patients and data collection

Three families with familial pheochromocytoma were evaluated for past medical history and complete physical examination in endocrine ward, Shariati hospital, Tehran University of Medical science. The case-notes and hospital databases were examined for additional required data. The tumor size was taken as the widest diameter recorded on pathological report or radiological, if the tumor had not been removed. Operative reports were reviewed to determine intra operative findings and types of surgical procedures. If there was evidence of extra-adrenal disease and if additional organ resection was necessary, specific notes were made.
All pheochromocyroms in this study were arising from the adrenal gland and no extra adrenal or paraganglioma was included. Adrenal bed recurrence was not a criterion for malignancy. The metastases were documented in all malignant cases. Metastatic disease was defined as evidence of distant spread in tissue not normally containing chromaffin tissue i.e. bone, liver, lung or lymph nodes.

2.1 Biochemical testing and localization studies

Routine biochemical tests, evaluation of 24 hours urine catecholamine metabolites, abdominal computed tomography (CT) or magnetic resonance imaging (MRI) and/or 131 Iodine_metaiodobenzylguanidine (MIBG) were done too. The malignant pheochromocytoma was diagnosed based on presence or absence of metastasis in radiological or pathological report.

2.2 Genetic analysis

2.2.1 RET proto-oncogene mutation screening

Genetic screening tests were done in family members. RET proto-oncogene mutation screening for exones 10, 11, 13 ,14, 15, 16 were examined by PCR and direct DNA sequencing. In patient 1, 4 and 5: Exons 10, 11, 13, 14, 15, and 16 RET proto-oncogene were examined by PCR and direct DNA sequencing (Alvandi et al., 2007).

2.2.2 VHL gene mutation screening

For VHL gene mutation screening, analysis of VHL gene was performed using Cruz et al protocol (Hasani-Ranjbar et al., 2009; Cruz et al., 2007). Exons 1, 2, 3 of VHL gene was amplified by PCR with the following primers:
1F - 5′ CCATCCTCTACCGAGCGCGCG 3′;
1R - 5′ GGGCTTCAGACCGTGCTATCG2;
3 F - 5′ TGCCCAGCCACCGGTGTG 2;
3 R - 5′ GTCTATCCTGTACTTACCACAACA;
3F - 5′ CACACTGCCACATACATGCACTC 3′;
3R - 5′ACTCATCAGTACCATCAAAAGCTG 3′.
Both forward and reverse strands were subjected to direct sequencing after PCR amplification. (Hasani-Ranjbar et al., 2009).

2.3 Protein modeling

The PDB file 1LM8 and 1VCB were used in the modeling work in order to find the potential impact of the residue mutation on the protein structure. NCBI blast module was used to determine the degree of residue conservation. *In silico* mutation was achieved with Swiss-

PdbViewer v.4 and minimization of the structure was done with the use of NOMAD-Ref server (http://lorentz.immstr.pasteur.fr/gromacs) (*Lindahl et al., 2006).*

3. Results

3.1 Family 1

The index patient was born to non related parents of Persian origin, Presented with thyroid nodule at the age of 48 years. His past medical history was unremarkable. He had no history of hypertensive crisis or headache. His daughter has had medullary thyroid cancer. And total thyroidectomy was done for her at the age of 23. Fine needle aspiration biopsy in the father was compatible with MTC and preoperational screening for pheochromocytoma was in favor of bilateral adrenal mass.

DNA was isolated from peripheral blood leucocytes using salting out method. Exones 10, 11, 13, 14, 15, 16 of RET proto-oncogene localized to 10q11.2 was examined by direct DNA sequencing. This resulted in identification of mutations in Exon 11, codon 634, TGC>CGC (Cystein>Arginine), which was indicative of hereditary MTC and Pheochromocytoma. The presence of this mutation was confirmed by sequencing of the complementary strand as well. This mutation was found in 2 other daughters and one of his sons and one of his nephews too.

One of the daughters (Figure 2, Patient 1) had thyroid nodule and complete evaluation was consistent with medulary thyroid cancer. Biochemical tests and radiological study for pheochromocytoma was done and the results were against adrenal mass. There was no evidence in favor of pheochromocytoma or Medullary thyroid cancer in three other RET proto-oncogen cariers. However total prophylactic thyroidectomy was done for all of them.

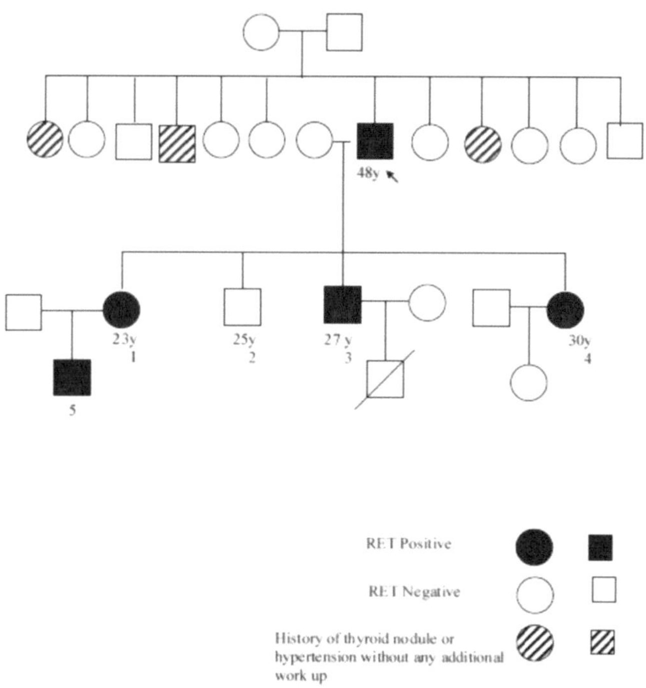

Fig. 2. Genetic relationship of multiple endocrine neoplasia type 2.

Bilateral adrenalectomy and then total thyroidectomy was done for the index patient (Figure 2, index patient). 2 years after bilateral adrenalectomy the patient presented with hypertention crisis and headache as he was on replacement therapy with prednisolon, Fludrocortisone and levothyroxine. Biochemical tests for pheochromocytoma and abdominal MRI was in favor of a 30 mm right adrenal mass. Evaluation for hyperparathyroidism was negative in all family members.

3.2 Family 2

Five sisters of Persian origin with grave clinical features of pheochromocytoma have been reported in our previous work (Hasani-Ranjbar et al, 2009). The index patient presented with cerebal hemorrhage and coma at the age of 29 years. After complete evaluation malignant metastatic pheochromocytoma confirmed and the patient was operated. Clinical manifestation of VHL, MEN syndrome and neurofibromatosis were negative in this patient and his family. Evaluation of other family members was consistent with malignant pheochromocytoma in four sisters. Bilateral adrenalectomy was done for them. 2 of these sisters died because of complication of pheochromocytoma.

3.2.1 Genetic analysis

Genetic analysis of VHL gene was in favor of this syndromic pheochromocytoma. Sequence analysis of VHL gene exons showed presence of a missense mutation (499C>T in exon 3).

3.2.2 Protein modeling

Arg 167 was found to be highly conserved among various species. Its mutation to tryptophan was observed to affect the hydrogen bondings of that residue within pVHL itself, and probably causing changes in the tertiary structure of the protein. *In silico* mutation of the residue and subsequent minimization of the Trp167 containing structure was performed and an overall RMSD of 0.519 A ° was obtained for the mutated structure with the use of backbone only, and 0.597 A ° with the use of all atoms. The most affected residue was found to be Leu 169 with RMSD of 1.902 (backbone) and 2.665 A °(all atoms). Figure 3 shows the position of Arg 167 in the pVHL tertiary structure (figure 3).

3.3 Family 3

A 45 year old man presented with abdominal pain and hypertension from 1 year ago. The patient was a known case of neurofibromatosis type 1 that presented at the age of 15 year with hyperpigmented and hypopigmented lesions in trunk, arms, feet and axillary areas. Family history was positive for neurofibromatosis in his mother and brother.

Biochemical tests and imaging was compatible with malignant pheochromocytoma. The size of mass was 120*70 mm. Left adrenalectomy and nephrectomy and splenectomy were done for him. After surgery the symptoms improved and blood pressure was controlled. The patient had poor compliance in follow up.

After 5 years he was admitted again for evaluation of hypertensive crisis. Again biochemical tests were consistent with pheochromocytoma and relapse. Imaging study and liver biopsy confirmed metastatic pheochromocytoma to liver and para-aortic area. 131I-MIBG therapy was done for him.

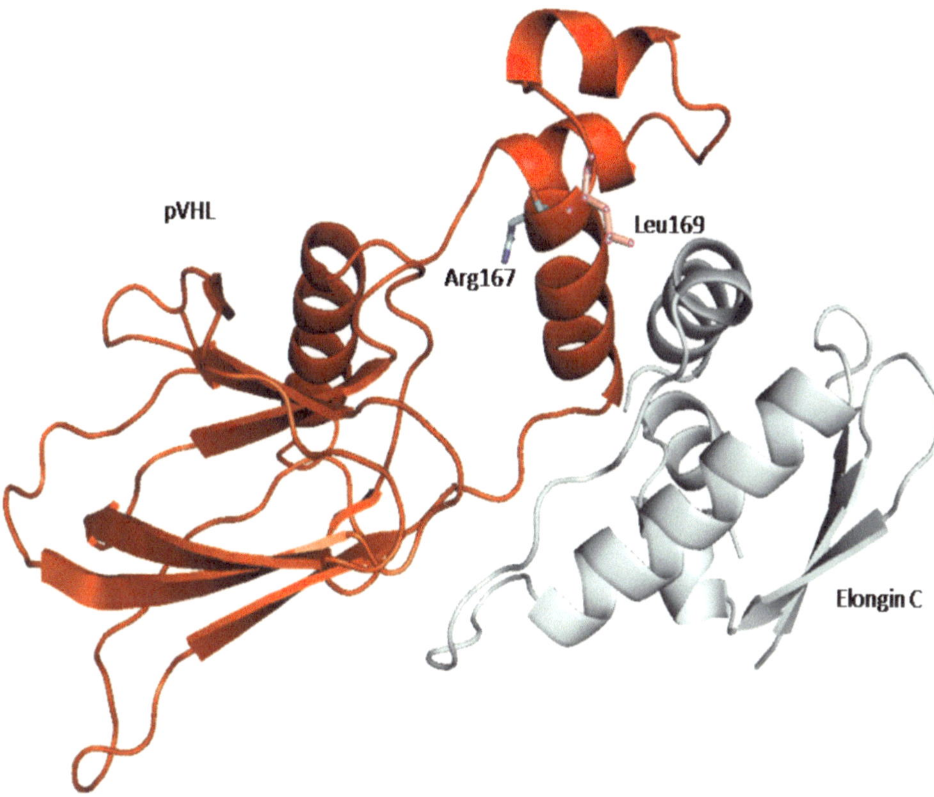

Fig. 3. pVHL (1LQB.PDB) is shown in cartoon representation, in the left part of the picture, interacting with Elongin C (right). The location of Arg 167 and Leu 169 residues is indicated with labels, and the residues are shown as sticks . Mutation of Arg 167 to Trp is suggested to affect both secondary and tertiary structure of pVHL. (This image has been created using PyMOL).

4. Discussion

Here we present three distinct families with intra adrenal pheochromocytoma (Table 2).

Subject	Family	Gender	Age at presentation	Clinical manifestation	Pheochromocytoma	Mutation	Treatment
1	1	M	48y	MTC	+	RET(codon 634, TGC>CGC	BilateralAdrenalectomy/Total thyroidectomy
2	1	F	23y	MTC	-	RET(codon 634, TGC>CGC	Total thyroidectomy
3	1	M	27y	No Symptom/No sign/MTC	-	RET(codon 634, TGC>CGC	Prophylactic Total thyroidectomy
4	1	F	30y	No Symptom/No Sign	-	RET(codon 634, TGC>CGC	Prophylactic Total thyroidectomy
5	1	M	2y	No Symptom/No Sign	-	RET(codon 634, TGC>CGC	Prophylactic Total thyroidectomy
6	2	F	29y	Cerebral Hemorrhage	+/Bilateral /Malignant	VHL Gene Mutation (499C>T)	Bilateral Adrenalectomy
7	2	F	23y	Malignant Hypertension	+/Malignant	Died on Operation	-
8	2	F	21y	Cerebral Hemorrhage	+/	Died before Operation	-
9	2	F	18y	Symptomatic and Hypertensive	+/Bilateral/malignant	VHL Gene Mutation (499C>T)	Bilateral Adrenalectomy
10	2	F	26y	Asymptomatic/biochemical tests+	+/Bilateral/Malignant	VHL Gene Mutation (499C>T)	Bilateral Adrenalectomy
11	3	M	50y	Hypertensive	+/Unilateral/Malignant	RET Negative VHL Negative	I131 MIBG Therapy

Abbreviations: VHL= von Hippel Lindau, MEN= multiple endocrine neoplasia, NF=Neurofibromatosis, Family 1=MEN2, Family 2= VHL, Family 3=NF, MTC=Medulary Thyroid Cancer, I131 MIBG = 131 Iodine_metaiodobenzylguanidine

Table 2. Genetic mutations and disease phenotype in the MEN 2, VHL and NF1 families.

4.1 Family 1

The index patient in family 1 who presented with thyroid nodule diagnosed as MEN 2 syndrome according to MTC and pheochromocytoma. The patient had no symptom or sign for pheochromocytoma. It is obviously known that when pheochromocytoma is associated with the multiple endocrine neoplasia type 2 (MEN2) syndrome, symptoms are present in only about one-half of patients and only one-third has hypertension (Pomares et al., 1998).

Evaluation for primary parathyroid hyperplasia was negative in him and his family. In addition no mucosal neuromas on the lips and tongue were detected. The patient had MEN2B phenotype. As we mentioned before, MEN2B shares the inherited predisposition to medullary thyroid cancer and pheochromocytoma that occurs in MEN2A. There are, however, important clinical differences. Patients with MEN2B tend to have mucosal neuromas and intestinal ganglioneuromas. Many of these patients have development abnormalities, a Marfanoid habitus, and myelinated corneal nerves. Furthermore, the tumor is often more aggressive and of earlier onset than in MEN2A; as a result, early diagnosis and prevention for other family members was very critical (Donovan et al., 1989; Mathew et al., 1987). Since MEN2B is caused by specific RET mutations we conducted genetic evaluation for categorization of the syndrome (MEN2A versus MEN2B) (Eng et al., 1996). The clinical feature was matched with MEN2B which is actually more aggressive. On the other hand genetic evaluation was consistent with a known mutation related to MEN2A in which prophylactic thyroidectomy is recommend to be done in carriers later. As we showed in results we identified mutations in Exon 11, codon 634, TGC>CGC (Cystein>Arginine), which was indicative of MEN2A syndrome.

The penetrance of hyperparathyroidism in those with mutations at this site is about 20 percent. Even with the same mutation the penetrance of hyperparathyroidism within families varies from 9 to 34 percent (Schunffenecker et al., 1998).

4.2 Family 2

Family 2 is an unusual form of VHL syndrome with malignant intra adrenal pheochromocytoma and retinal angioma diagnosed as VHL type 2. Clinical manifestation of VHL, MEN syndrome and neurofibromatosis were negative in index patient and his family up to 9 years when retinal angioma was detected. All clinical manifestation and genetic and protein modeling methods have been described in our previous work which published in familial cancer journal (Hasani-Ranjbar et al., 2009).

In this paper we reported the presence of a novel single nucleotide mutation in exon 3 of VHL gene c499 C>T causing substitution of Arginine by Tryptophan at position 167 (R 167 W) (Hasani-Ranjbar et al., 2009). This family has been followed for at least 9 years as RET negative isolated familial pheochromocytoma, finally diagnosed as VHL disease according to retinal angioma and VHL gene mutation. As we noted before malignant pheochromocytoma is very rare in VHL disease and other familial forms of pheochromocytoma.

Although clinical criteria were originally developed for the diagnosis of VHL based upon the finding of more than one VHL-associated tumor, now detection of a germline mutation in the VHL gene is typically used to establish the diagnosis, particularly in patients with a single manifestation of the condition (Lonser et al., 2003).

On average about 10 to 20% of patients with VHL disease develop pheochromocytoma, but this incidence varies dramatically from family to family depending on the specific mutation (Koch et al., 2002; Karsdrop et al., 1994; Lamiell et al., 1989; Linehan et al., 1995)

In pheochromocytoma associated with von Hippel-Lindau disease, 35 percent of patients have no symptoms, a normal blood pressure, and normal laboratory values for fractionated catecholamines and metanephrines (Walter et al., 1999b). In our report all patients had aggressive disease and only one of the family members was asymptomatic diagnosed as adrenal pheochromocytoma based on screening tests (Table2)(Hasani-Ranjbar et al., 2009). Malignant pheochromocytomas are histologically and biochemically the same as benign ones. The only reliable clue to the presence of a malignant pheochromocytoma is local invasion or distant metastases, which may occur as long as 20 years after resection (Goldstein et al., 1999; Pattarino & Bouloux 1996).

A recent study showed high risk factors predictive factors of malignant pheochromocytoma include, large (5 cm or greater) or heavy (250 gm or greater) tumors, multifocal and extra-adrenal tumors, early onset postoperative hypertension and higher plasma or urine metadrenaline (Feng et al., 2011). An initial report suggests that inhibin/activin beta-B subunit expression may help distinguish between benign and malignant disease; expression was strong or moderate in almost all benign adrenal pheochromocytomas (Salmenkivi et al., 2001). Also, expression of the 3 angiogenesis or metastasis related genes VEGF, Cox-2 and MVD helps determine the diagnosis of malignancy and suggests strict followup (Gimenez-Roqueplo et al., 2003; Brouwers et al., 2006).

4.2.1 Protein modeling

pVHL makes interactions with Elongin B and C, as well as HIF. The H1 helix of pVHL , where Arg 167 is located, is the interface between this protein and Elongin C, and a place where missense mutations occur frequently (Stebbinset et al., 1999). It seems that Arg 167 is involved in the correct positioning of the H1 helix, and that its mutation can also affect the hydrophobic interactions of Leu 168 with neighbour residues of Elongin C. the overall result is the disruption of some pVHL interactions with Elongin C (Figure 3).

4.3 Family 3

Family 3 is a kindred with neurofibromatosis and a member (A 45 year old man) with hypertension diagnosed as malignant pheochromocytoma. Hypertension is a frequent finding in adults with NF1 and may develop during childhood but pheochromocytoma is a much less common etiology. In these patients, the catecholamine-secreting tumor is usually a solitary benign adrenal pheochromocytoma, occasionally bilateral adrenal pheochromocytoma, and rarely a peri adrenal abdominal paraganglioma . Although neurofibromatosis type 1 as an autosomal dominant disorder is the most common familial cancer syndrome predisposing to pheochromocytoma, the risk of pheochromocytoma in this disorder is about 1% (Huson et al 1989; Riccardi et al., 1991).

Pheochromocytomas in patients with neurofibromatosis type 1 occur at the fifth decade. Our patient was a 45 years old man with an unusual presentation of pheochromocytma. Currently, except for the presence of the *SDHB* mutation, large size or an extra-adrenal location of the primary tumor, there are no reliable markers for predicting a high likelihood of developing metastatic disease. Pheochromocytoma in neurofibromatosis is usually benign and unilateral. Based on genetic background our expectation before surgery was a benign non metastatic tumor. As we mentioned before, the patient had a metastatic tumor and after 5 years metastasis to liver and para-aortic lymph nodes deteriorated the clinical course of disease. It seems to us that large mass (as detected in this patient firstly) beside local invasion is a critical predicting factor to malignancy and may have the highest impact for detecting metastasis in future.

At first we treated the patient with surgical resection of the adrenal mass, but in follow up for treatment of distance metastasis the only available modality was MIBG therapy. Considering positive MIBG scan we predicted that the tumor could up take iodine. To date, beside surgery, 131I-MIBG therapy is the single most valuable therapy for malignant pheochromocytomas. Results of a phase II trial using high dose I131 MIBG demonstrated 22% partial or complete response and 35% of patients having some degree of response (i.e. biochemical) without demonstrated progressive disease (Gonias et al.,2009). For future our plan could be chemoembolization of the liver if there is persistent disease.

5. Acknowledgment

We thank all the VHL, MEN and NF families and patients.

6. References

Alvandi, E., Pedram, M., Soroush, A.R., Noori Naier, B., Akrami, S.M. (2007), Detection of RET Proto-oncogene Cys634Arg Mutation, the Cause of Medullary Thyroid Carcinoma, in an Iranian Child. *Iran J Pediatr Suppl*,2, 301

Brandi, M.L., Gagel, R.F., Angeli, A., Bilezikian, J.P., Beck-Peccoz, P., Bordi, C., Conte-Devolx, B., Falchetti, A., Gheri, R.G., Libroia, A., Lips, C.J., Lombardi, G., Mannelli, M., Pacini, F., Ponder, B.A., Raue, F., Skogseid, B., Tamburrano, G., Thakker, R.V., Thompson, N.W., Tomassetti, P., Tonelli, F., Wells, S.A. Jr., Marx, S.J., (2001),Guidelines for diagnosis and therapy of MEN type 1 and type 2. *J Clin Endocrinol Metab*, 86,12,5658.

Brouwers, F.M., Eisenhofer, G., Tao, J.J., Kant, J.A., Adams, K.T., Linehan, W.M., Pacak, K.,(2006), High frequency of SDHB germline mutations in patients with malignant catecholamine-producing paragangliomas: implications for genetic testing. *J Clin Endocrinol Metab*,91,11,4505.

Carlson, K.M., Dou, S., Chi, D., Scavarda, N., Toshima, K., Jackson, C.E., Wells, S.A. Jr., Goodfellow, P.J., Donis-Keller, H., (1994),Single missense mutation in the tyrosine kinase catalytic domain of the RET protooncogene is associated with multiple endocrine neoplasia type 2B, *Proc Natl Acad Sci U S A, 91,4,1579-83.*

Ciotti, P., Garuti, A., Gulli, R., Ballestrero, A., Bellone ,E., Mandich, P.,(2009), Germline mutations in the von Hippel-Lindau gene in Italian patients. *Eur J Med Genet.*,52,5,311-4. Epub 2009 May 21.

Cruz, J.B., Fernandes, L.P., Clara, S.A., Conde, S.J., Perone, D., Kopp, P., Nogueira, C.R., (2007), Molecular analysis of the Von Hippel-Lindau (VHL) gene in a family with non-syndromic pheochromocytoma: the importance of genetic testing. *Arq Bras Endocrinol Metabol* , 51,1463-1467.

Donovan, D.T., Levy, M.L., Furst, E.J., Alford, B.R., Wheeler, T., Tschen, J.A., Gagel, R.F, (1989),Familial cutaneous lichen amyloidosis in association with multiple endocrine neoplasia type 2A: a new variant. *Henry Ford Hosp Med J*,37,3-4,147.

Dluhy, R.G.,(2002), Pheochromocytoma--death of an axiom. *N Engl J Med,* 346,19,1486.

Elder, E.E., G. Elder, and C. Larsson, (2005),Pheochromocytoma and functional paraganglioma syndrome: no longer the 10% tumor. *J Surg Oncol*, 89,3, 193-201.

Eng, C., Clayton, D., Schuffenecker, I., Lenoir, G., Cote, G., Gagel, R.F., van Amstel, H.K., Lips, C.J., Nishisho, I., Takai, S.I., Marsh, D.J., Robinson, B.G., Frank-Raue, K., Raue, F., Xue, F., Noll, W.W., Romei, C., Pacini, F., Fink, M., Niederle, B., Zedenius, J., Nordenskjöld, M., Komminoth, P., Hendy, G.N., Mulligan, L.M.,(1996), The relationship between specific RET proto-oncogene mutations and disease phenotype in multiple endocrine neoplasia type 2. International RET mutation consortium analysis. *JAMA*,276,19,1575.

Eng, C., Guillausseau, P.J., Lenoir, G.M., (1998),Risk and penetrance of primary hyperparathyroidism in multiple endocrine neoplasia type 2A families with mutations at codon 634 of the RET proto-oncogene. Groupe D'etude des Tumeurs à Calcitonine. *J Clin Endocrinol Metab*,83,2,487.

Feldkamp, M.M., Gutmann, D.H., Guha, A.,(1998), Neurofibromatosis type 1: piecing the puzzle together. *Can J Neurol Sci*, 25,3,181.

Feng, F., Zhu, Y., Wang, X., Wu, Y., Zhou, W., Jin, X., Zhang, R., Sun, F., Kasoma, Z., Shen, Z. (2011),Predictive Factors for Malignant Pheochromocytoma: Analysis of 136 Patients.*J Urol*, Mar 16

Gonias, S., Goldsby, R., Matthay, K.K., Hawkins, R., Price, D., Huberty, J., Damon, L., Linker, C., Sznewajs, A., Shiboski, S., Fitzgerald, P.,(2009), Phase II study of high-dose [131I]metaiodobenzylguanidine therapy for patients with metastatic pheochromocytoma and paraganglioma. *J Clin Oncol* ,1,27,25,4162-8. Epub 2009 Jul 27

Gimenez-Roqueplo, A.P., Favier, J., Rustin, P., Rieubland, C., Crespin, M., Nau, V., Khau, Van Kien, P., Corvol, P., Plouin, P.F., Jeunemaitre, X., (2003),COMETE Network ,Mutations in the SDHB gene are associated with extra-adrenal and/or malignant phaeochromocytomas. *Cancer Res*,63,17,5615.

Goldstein, R.E., O'Neill, J.A. Jr., Holcomb, G.W. 3rd, Morgan, W.M. 3rd, Neblett, W.W. 3rd, Oates, J.A., Brown, N., Nadeau, J., Smith, B., Page, D.L., Abumrad, N.N., Scott, H.W. Jr.,(1999), Clinical experience over 48 years with pheochromocytoma. *Ann Surg*,229,6,755-64; discussion 764-6

Gomy, I., Molfetta, G.A., de Andrade Barreto, E., Ferreira, C.A., Zanette, D.L., Casali-da-Rocha, J.C., Silva, W.A. Jr.(2010), Clinical and molecular characterization of Brazilian families with von Hippel-Lindau disease: a need for delineating genotype-phenotype correlation. *Fam Cancer,* 2010 ,9,4,635-42.

Hasani-Ranjbar, S., Amoli, M.M., Ebrahim-Habibi, A., Haghpanah,V., Hejazi, M., Soltani, A., Larijani, B.,(2009), Mutation screening of VHL gene in a family with malignant bilateral pheochromocytoma: from isolated familial pheochromocytoma to von Hippel-Lindau disease. *Fam Cancer*,8,4,465-71. Epub 2009 Aug 1.

Hasani-Ranjbar, S., Amoli, M.M., Ebrahim-Habibi, A., Gozashti, M.H., Khalili, N., Sayyahpour, F.A., Hafeziyeh, J., Soltani, A., Larijani, B.,(2010), A new frameshift MEN1 gene mutation associated with familial malignant insulinomas. *Fam Cancer,* Dec 24.

Hachen, R., Barnicoat, A., Li, H., Wallace, P., Van Biervliet, J.P., Stevenson ,D., Viskochil, D., Baralle, D., Haan, E., Riccardi, V., Turnpenny, P., Lazaro, C., Messiaen, L., (2007),An absence of cutaneous neurofibromas associated with a 3-bp inframe deletion in exon 17 of the NF1 gene (c.2970-2972 delAAT): evidence of a clinically significant NF1 genotype-phenotype correlation. *Am J Hum Genet*, 80,1,140.

Huson, S.M., Compston, D.A., Clark, P., Harper, P.S., (1989),A genetic study of von Recklinghausen neurofibromatosis in south east Wales. I. Prevalence, fitness, mutation rate, and effect of parental transmission on severity, *J Med Genet, 26,11, 704-11.*

Kantorovich, V., King, K.S., Pacak, K.,(2010), SDH-related pheochromocytoma and paraganglioma. *Best Pract Res Clin Endocrinol Metab*,24,3,415-24.

Karsdorp, N., et al., Von Hippel-Lindau disease: new strategies in early detection and treatment. Am J Med, 1994. 97(2): p. 158-68.

Koch, C.A., Huang, S.C., Zhuang, Z., Stolle, C., Azumi, N., Chrousos, G.P., Vortmeyer, A.O., Pacak, K., *(2002),*Somatic VHL gene deletion and point mutation in MEN 2A-associated pheochromocytoma. *Oncogene,* 21,3, 479-82.

Kim, W.Y., Kaelin, W.G. (2004) Role of VHL gene mutation in human cancer. *J Clin Oncol,* 22, 4991-5004 .

Lammert, M., Friedman, J.M., Kluwe, L., Mautner, V.F.,(2005),Prevalence of neurofibromatosis 1 in German children at elementary school enrollment. *Arch Dermatol,*141,1,71.

Lamiell, J.M., Salazar F.G., & Hsia Y.E. (1989*),* von Hippel-Lindau disease affecting 43 members of a single kindred. *Medicine (Baltimore),* 68,1, 1-29.

Linehan, W., Lerman, M. & Zbar,B., (1995),Identification of the VHL Gene: Its Role in Renal Carcinoma, *JAMA,* 273, 564-570.

Ledbetter, D.H., Rich, D.C., O'Connell, P., Leppert, M., Carey, J.C., (1989),Precise localization of NF1 to 17q11.2 by balanced translocation. *Am J Hum Genet,* 44,1,20.

Lenders, J.W., Eisenhofer, G., Mannelli, M., Pacak, K., (2005),Phaeochromocytoma. *Lancet.,* 20-26,366(9486),665-75.

Lindahl ,E., Azuara, C., Koehl, P., Delarue, M., (2006) NOMAD-Ref: visualization, deformation and refinement of macromolecular structures based on all-atom normal mode analysis. *Nucleic Acids Res,* 34,W52–W56].

Lonser, R.R., Glenn, G.M., Walther, M., Chew, E.Y., Libutti, S.K., Linehan, W.M., Oldfield, E.H. (2003),von Hippel-Lindau disease. *Lancet,*361,9374,2059.

López-Jiménez, E., Gómez-López, G., Leandro-García, L.J., Muñoz, I., Schiavi, F., Montero-Conde, C., de Cubas, A.A., Ramires, R., Landa, I., Leskelä, S., Maliszewska, A., Inglada-Pérez, L., de la Vega, L., Rodríguez-Antona , C., Letón, R., Bernal, C., de Campos, J.M., Diez-Tascón, C., Fraga, M.F., Boullosa, C., Pisano, D.G., Opocher, G., Robledo, M., Cascón, A. (2010),Research resource: Transcriptional profiling reveals different pseudohypoxic signatures in SDHB and VHL-related pheochromocytomas. *Mol Endocrinol.* 24,12,2382-91. Epub 2010 Oct 27.

Mathew, C.G., Chin, K.S., Easton, D.F., Thorpe, K., Carter, C., Liou, G.I., Fong, S.L., Bridges, C.D., Haak, H., Kruseman, A.C.,(1987), A linked genetic marker for multiple endocrine neoplasia type 2A on chromosome 10. *Nature,* 328,6130,527.

Manger., W.M.,& Gifford, R.W., (2002),Pheochromocytoma. *J Clin Hypertens,* 4,1, 62-72.

Mulligan, L.M., Eng, C., Healey, C.S., Clayton, D., Kwok, J.B., Gardner, E., Ponder, M.A., Frilling, A., Jackson, C.E., Lehnert, H., (1994),Specific mutations of the RET proto-oncogene are related to disease phenotype in MEN 2A and FMTC. *Nat Genet,*6,1,70.

Neumann, H.P., Bausch, B., McWhinney, S.R., Bender, B.U., Gimm, O., Franke, G., Schipper, J., Klisch, J., Altehoefer, C., Zerres, K., Januszewicz, A., Eng, C., Smith, W.M., Munk, R., Manz, T., Glaesker, S., Apel, T.W., Treier, M., Reineke, M., Walz, M.K., Hoang-Vu, C., Brauckhoff, M., Klein-Franke, A., Klose, P., Schmidt, H., Maier-Woelfle, M., Peçzkowska, M., Szmigielski, C., Eng, C., Freiburg-Warsaw-Columbus (2002),Pheochromocytoma Study Group, Germ-line mutations in nonsyndromic pheochromocytoma. *N Engl J Med,*346,19,1459.

Neumann, H.P., Berger, D.P., Sigmund, G., Blum, U., Schmidt, D., Parmer, R.J., Volk, B., Kirste, G., (1993),Pheochromocytomas, multiple endocrine neoplasia type 2, and von Hippel-Lindau disease. *N Engl J Med,*329,21,1531.

North, K. (1993), Neurofibromatosis type 1: review of the first 200 patients in an Australian clinic. *J Child Neurol.* 8,4,395.

O'Riordain, D.S., Young, W.F. Jr., Grant, C.S., Carney, J.A., van Heerden, J.A., (1996),Clinical spectrum and outcome of functional extraadrenal paraganglioma. *World J Surg, 20,7, 916-21.*

Pacak, K., Ilias, I., Adams, K.T., Eisenhofer, G., (2005),Biochemical diagnosis, localization and management of pheochromocytoma: focus on multiple endocrine neoplasia type 2 in relation to other hereditary syndromes and sporadic forms of the tumour. *J Intern Med, 2005,* 257,1,60-8.

Pattarino, F., Bouloux, P.M. (1996),The diagnosis of malignancy in phaeochromocytoma. *Clin Endocrinol (Oxf),* 44,239.

Patocs ,A., Gergics, P., Balogh, K., Toth, M., Fazakas, F., Liko, I., Racz, K., (2008) Ser80Ile mutation and a concurrent Pro25Leu variant of the VHL gene in an extended Hungarian von Hippel-Lindau family,*BMC Med Genet* ,9, 29.

Pomares, F.J., Cañas, R., Rodriguez, J.M., Hernandez, A.M., Parrilla, P., Tebar, F.J., (1998),Differences between sporadic and multiple endocrine neoplasia type 2A phaeochromocytoma. *Clin Endocrinol (Oxf),* 48,195.

Riccardi, V.M., *(1991),*Neurofibromatosis: past, present, and future. *N Engl J Med, 324,18, 1283-5.*

Salmenkivi, K., Arola, J., Voutilainen, R., Ilvesmäki, V., Haglund ,C., Kahri, A.I., Heikkilä, P., Liu, J., (2001),Inhibin/activin betaB-subunit expression in pheochromocytomas favors benign diagnosis.*J Clin Endocrinol Metab*,86,5,2231.

Schuffenecker, I., Virally-Monod, M., Brohet, R., Goldgar, D., Conte-Devolx, B., Leclerc, L., Chabre, O., Boneu, A., Caron, J., Houdent, C., Modigliani, E., Rohmer, V., Schlumberger, M.,

Shen, M.H., Harper, P.S., Upadhyaya, M.,(1996), Molecular genetics of neurofibromatosis type 1 (NF1). *J Med Genet*,33,1,2.

Upadhyaya, M., Huson, S.M., Davies, M., Thomas, N., Chuzhanova, N., Giovannini, S., Evans, D.G., Howard, E., Kerr, B., Griffiths, S., Consoli, C., Side, L., Adams, D., Pierpont, M.,

Strong, V.E., Kennedy, T., Al-Ahmadie, H., Tang, L., Coleman, J., Fong, Y., Brennan, M., Ghossein, R.A., (2008),Prognostic indicators of malignancy in adrenal pheochromocytomas: clinical, histopathologic, and cell cycle/apoptosis gene expression analysis. *Surgery*,143,6,759-68. Epub 2008 Apr 14.

Stebbins, C.E., Kaelin, W.G., Pavlevitch, N.P., (1999) Structure of the VHL-ElonginC-ElonginB complex: implications for VHL tumor suppressor function. *Science,* 284:455–46].

Walther, M.M., Herring, J., Enquist, E., Keiser, H.R., Linehan, W.M., (1999a),von Recklinghausen's disease and pheochromocytomas. *J Urol*,162,5,1582.

Walther, M.M., Reiter, R., Keiser, H.R., Choyke, P.L., Venzon, D., Hurley, K., Gnarra, J.R., Reynolds, J.C., Glenn, G.M., Zbar, B., Linehan, W.M.,(1999b), Clinical and genetic characterization of pheochromocytoma in von Hippel-Lindau families: comparison with sporadic pheochromocytoma gives insight into natural history of pheochromocytoma. *J Urol*,162,3 ,(Pt 1),659-64.

Whalen, R.K., Althausen, A.F., Daniels, G.H. *(1992),* Extra-adrenal pheochromocytoma. *J Urol,* 147, 1-10.

Zbar, B., Kishida, T., Chen, F., Schmidt, L., Maher, E.R., Richards, F.M., Crossey, P.A., Webster, A.R., Affara, N.A., Ferguson-Smith, M.A., Brauch, H., Glavac, D., Neumann, H.P., Tisherman, S., Mulvihill, J.J., Gross, D.J., Shuin, T., Whaley, J., Seizinger, B., Kley, N., Olschwang, S., Boisson, C., Richard, S., Lips, C.H., Lerman, M.,(1996), Germline mutations in the Von Hippel-Lindau disease (VHL) gene in families from North America, Europe, and Japan. *Hum Mutat*,8,4,348.